A Colour Atlas of Diabetes
(Second edition)

A Colour Atlas of

Diabetes

Second Edition

Arnold Bloom
MD, FRCP
Honorary Consultant Physician
Whittington Hospital
London

John Ireland
MD, FRCP (Ed)
Late Consultant Physician
Southern General Hospital
Glasgow

With revisions by
Peter Watkins
MD, FRCP
Physician in Charge, Diabetic Department
King's College Hospital
London

Wolfe Publishing Ltd

Copyright © Wolfe Publishing Ltd, 1992
First published 1980, by Wolfe Publishing Ltd
Second edition published 1992
Printed by Smeets-Weert, Holland
ISBN 0 7234 0972 2

A CIP catalogue record for this book is available from the British Library.

This book is one of the titles in the series of
Wolfe Medical Atlases, a series that brings together
the world's largest systematic published collection of
diagnostic colour photographs.

For a full list of Atlases in the series, plus forthcoming
titles and details of our surgical, dental and veterinary
Atlases, please write to Wolfe Medical Publications Ltd,
Brook House, 2-16 Torrington Place, London WC1E 7LT, England.

Contents

Acknowledgements

We are indebted to many friends and colleagues who contributed illustrations for this text. In particular we acknowledge the help of Drs A Dick, G H Roberts and Mr G F Headden in preparing, staining and photographing most of the histology; Dr Georgina McCreath provided much of the radiology and Dr J Williamson contributed extensively to the ophthalmology. Other colleagues in Glasgow who gave material include Drs A D Beattie, D Doyle, A A M Gibson, K W Grossart, A C MacCuish, and N W Morley. The late Prof. A G Cudworth and his colleagues Drs A Gorsuch, D Hodge and Eva Wolf, St Bartholomew's Hospital gave the HLA illustrations; Professors S Bloom and Julia Polak, Hammersmith Hospital provided the pancreatic electron micrographs and the immuno-peroxidase stained islet tissue and Dr C Mallinson the glucagonoma pictures. Professor P K Thomas and Dr R H M King and Dr P J Watkins, London; Drs J D Ward and W R Timperley, Sheffield and Drs D J Ewing, I W Campell and B F Clarke, Edinburgh gave material mainly in the neurology section. Mr R G Law, Whittington Hospital contributed the fetal and ultrasound pictures and Drs J Terpstra and J Ruys of Leiden the Xrays of fetal abnormalities. The scanning electron micrographs of the glomerulus are the work of P M Rowles and Dr Patricia McLean, the Bland-Sutton and Courtauld Institutes, London, the transmission electron micrographs were made by Miss Sharida Abrahams, Glasgow. The radiographs of renal papillary necrosis are by courtesy of Dr F G Adams, Glasgow and the editor of 'Clinical Radiology'. The histopathology pictures on a normal islet and a similarly-stained islet from a child who died from ketoacidosis appear with the permission of Dr Gian Franco Bottazo of the Middlesex Hospital. These pictures originally appeared in his article 'Death of a beta cell: homicide or suicide?' in *Diabetic Medicine*, with the kind permission of Dr A Foulis, Glasgow.

Preface

Diabetes is a common and widespread disorder occurring in every part of the world. The inception of insulin therapy over 70 years ago has enabled diabetic patients to live a full life. In their later years they often suffer degenerative complications, particularly vascular disorders, kidney disease, neuropathy and blindness. Indeed, no system is unaffected by diabetes. The study of this disorder, therefore, involves almost every aspect of medicine and pathology.

In this Second Edition we have taken the opportunity to add further illustrations, and to enhance the text, particularly by the addition of the new chapter on Management.

The purpose of the book remains to present in graphic form the clinical and histological manifestations of diabetes. It is hoped in this way, it will prove of practical value to the medical student, the house physician and the general practitioner who wish to gain a better understanding of this disorder.

1 History

Diabetes has been known to mankind since antiquity. Thus a disorder with 'honeyed urine' appears in ancient Sanskrit literature, while the Egyptian papyrus of Ebers dating from 1550 BC contains dietary remedies for those passing abundant urine. The first clear clinical account of diabetes is given in the writings of Aretaeus the Cappodocian (AD 170) who described 'this mysterious affection . . . being a melting down of flesh and limbs into urine . . . life is short, disgusting and painful, thirst unquenchable, death inevitable . . .' To this day we remain unable to challenge his observation that diabetes is a mysterious disease.

Thomas Cawley was the first to hint at pancreatic involvement in diabetes. Writing in the *London Medical Journal* of 1788 he described a case of diabetes which, at autopsy, showed marked pancreatic damage and led Cawley to postulate that pancreatic disease might be causally related to diabetes. The importance of the pancreas was established by Oskar Minkowski in 1889, who described, with Von Mering, how pancreatectomy made a laboratory dog urinate excessively and how the urine attracted flies (5). In a moment of inspiration he tested the urine for sugar and found large amounts present.

Twenty years earlier, Paul Langerhans, while still a medical student, wrote a treatise on the pancreas which included the first clear description of the islet tissues now bearing his name. Although the significance of the islets escaped Langerhans, Gustave Laguesse (1893) suggested that they might produce an endocrine secretion. After the development of the concept of hormones by Ernest Starling (1904), workers in Germany, Roumania and elsewhere were concentrating their attention on extracting insulin from the pancreas. The Canadian surgeon Frederick Banting working with the medical student Charles Best in the summer of 1921, were the first to succeed in reaching this objective. They showed that their pancreatic extract lowered the blood glucose in dogs who had been made diabetic by pancreatectomy (6).

The discovery of insulin, one of the greatest triumphs of twentieth century medicine, was quickly translated into a lifesaving remedy. Thanks to the work of James Bertram Collip and the pharmaceutical industry, insulin (4) became available for clinical care throughout the world within 2 years of Banting's and Best's work. In Britain,

R.D. Lawrence who was himself a diabetic, and among the first to receive insulin, became one the world's leading diabetic physicians; his book, *The Diabetic Life*, provided many generations of diabetic patients with much needed and very shrewd practical advice.

Although a new era had dawned for the diabetic patient, there remained problems to be surmounted.

Paul Kimmelstiel, an astute German pathologist, noted at autopsy curious nodular lesions in the glomeruli of diabetics. Other pathologists were sceptical, at first, when his findings were published with the help of Clifford Wilson in 1936 (1). However, within a few years several more renal vascular lesions were noted in diabetics. Interest had also been awakened in diabetic retinopathy (Ballantyne and Loewenstein, 1944) and the concept of a specific and widespread diabetic small blood vessel disease, affecting especially the kidneys and retina was postulated by Knud Lundbaek (1954). It became apparent, therefore, that the price of survival bought with insulin for the diabetic was a life shortened and crippled by degenerative vascular disease. Although there was no question that insulin was a safe and natural hormone, the troubles of repeated injections and the risks of hypoglycaemia led to the search for an oral substitute. The mildly hypoglycaemic effect of salicylates had been known since the late nineteenth century. It was, however, the hypoglycaemic side-effect of sulphonamides discovered during a typhoid epidemic in southwest France in 1940 by Marcel Jambon that led to the development of the hypoglycaemic sulphonylureas. Auguste Loubatière investigated this side-effect and demonstrated its dependence upon an intact pancreas. The search then began for the sulphonylurea best able to stimulate the beta-cell without serious side-effects. Franke and Fuchs (1954) working in Germany were the first to produce a safe and effective oral agent. Since then many improvements have been made, so that today a wide range of such drugs is available proving a boon to many diabetics—especially the elderly—who might otherwise have required insulin injections.

Although these therapeutic advances with insulin and oral agents have made it possible to control diabetic symptoms, they have failed to prevent the serious vascular and other complications of diabetes. Thus the search continues for the fundamental causes of diabetes and its complications. Research has centred upon the rôle of insulin. An understanding of the basic amino acid structure of insulin was made possible by the work of Frederick Sanger (1958) in Cambridge, while more recently its three-dimensional structure has been elucidated by Dorothy Hodgkin using Xray crystallography. Both researchers, like the discoverer of insulin, have received Nobel prizes for their work. The major advance in our understanding of blood levels of insulin (and other hormones) stemmed from the development of immunoassay techniques by Berson and Yalow (1962). The first step towards determining the sequence of pancreatic insulin synthesis was made by the discovery of pro-insulin and its C-peptide by Donald Steiner in 1967. Now a host of pancreatic, gut and other hormones have been

recognised, each having a part to play in either aiding or hindering the action of insulin.

With a rapid growth of interest in autoimmunity, insulin antibodies and HLA associations, much work still remains to be done. Today a child who develops diabetes can lead a full and happy life with insulin treatment. His expectation of life ahead, however, is considerably reduced and his later years may be clouded by ill health and blindness. Until we can recognise the cause and prevention of these degenerative changes, continued effort and research will be needed. Best of all, the day may dawn when we can recognise those who are susceptible to diabetes and then be able to prevent its occurrence.

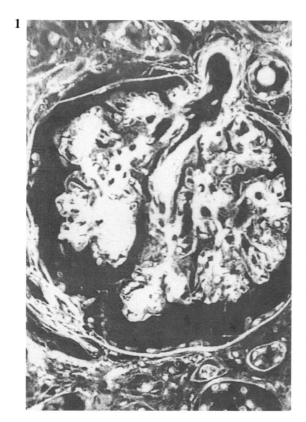

1 **Nodular diabetic glomerulosclerosis:** one of the illustrations from the original description of this condition by Kimmelstiel and Wilson in 1936.

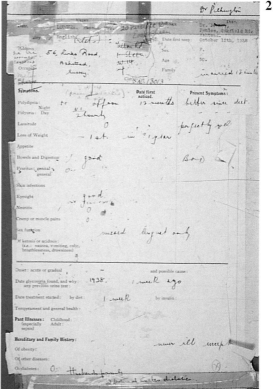

2 **A patient's record in the hand of Dr R.D. Lawrence of King's College Hospital,** dated 1938. Dr Lawrence, who was himself diabetic, first received insulin in May 1923. He established the Diabetic Department at King's College Hospital, played a leading role in forming the British Diabetic Association in 1934, and was later made President of the International Diabetic Federation.

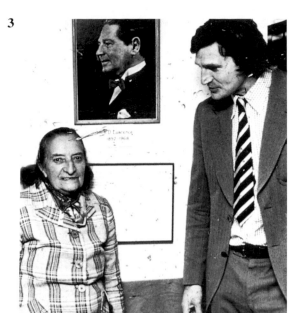

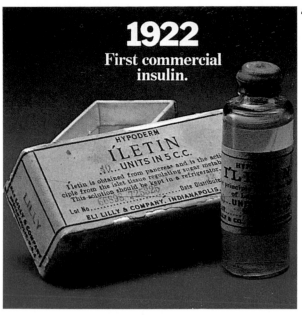

3 Miss Pearce, secretary to Dr R.D. Lawrence for many years, with one of his sons (right) Dr Adam Lawrence. Note photograph of Dr R.D. Lawrence in the background.

4 First commercial insulin (Iletin) manufactured by Eli Lilly in 1922. (*Reproduced with kind permission from* Eli Lilly & Co.)

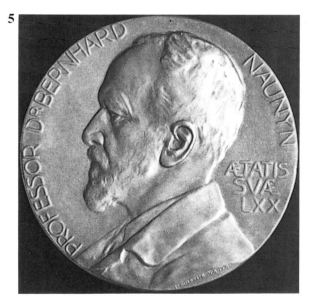

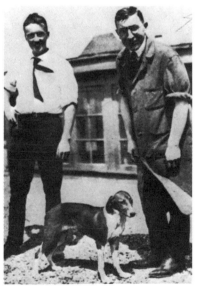

5 Dr Bernard Naunyn, physician (1839-1925) in whose Strasbourg laboratories Von Mering and Minkowski made their crucial observation in a dog that pancreatectomy causes diabetes. Naunyn wrote an important textbook on diabetes (*Der Diabetes Mellitus*, (1898) and a very instructive autobiography (*Erinnerungen Gedanken und Meinungen des Dr B. Naunyn*, 1925).

6 Frederick Banting and Charles Best with the first dog to receive insulin by injection.

2 Clinical presentation and aetiology

Diabetes mellitus can be defined as a chronic disorder characterised by a raised level of glucose in the blood. Since there are many factors which can influence blood glucose, diabetes can be the outcome of many different causes, some hereditary, some environmental and some hormonal. Diabetes is no more a single disease than is anaemia and a better understanding of the aetiology is a necessary prerequisite for intelligent management.

From the clinical viewpoint, the aetiology of the commonest forms of diabetes is unknown and they are sometimes referred to as primary diabetes. These include: type I or insulin-dependent diabetes mellitus (IDDM); type II or non-insulin-dependent diabetes mellitus (NIDDM); and the much rarer types of diabetes usually associated with other hereditary disorders. The causes of some forms of diabetes are known and they are therefore classified as secondary diabetes. These include diabetes due to destruction of the pancreas by drugs, disease or surgery and diabetes due to hormonal imbalance.

Primary diabetes

Type I diabetes (insulin dependent)

This type of diabetes starts most commonly in children or young adults, but it may occur at any age, often in the very elderly (**Table 2**). It is characterised by the rapid onset of symptoms especially thirst, polyuria and lassitude. There is usually considerable loss of weight and most diabetics of this type are underweight at diagnosis. Occasionally, however, type I diabetes can occur in the overweight. Other common symptoms include blurring of vision, paraesthesiae, cramp in the muscles, pruritus vulvae and balanitis. The urine, at diagnosis, contains sugar and significant amounts of acetone, while blood examination reveals evidence of dehydration (a raised urea and haematocrit), a tendency to ketoacidosis and a blood glucose exceeding 11.1mmol/1 (200mg/100dl). Estimation of plasma insulin shows the levels to be low and responding poorly, or not at all, to an oral or intravenous glucose load. In essence, then, type I diabetics are suffering from insulin deprivation and most of the metabolic disorders stem from this deficiency. However, lack of insulin may not be the only defect. Excess of glucagon and pancreatic polypeptide can also be demonstrated and these may be additional factors in the pathogenesis of diabetes of this type, which will be discussed further on.

Type I diabetics need insulin to live, for without it the symptoms worsen, drowsiness gives place to increasing ketoacidosis and fatal coma. Hence, these patients are referred to as insulin dependent.

Inheritance

About 10 per cent of children who develop diabetes have a sibling or parent with the disorder, whereas only 1 per cent of non-diabetic children have a diabetic relative. Two conclusions emerge. First, there is undoubtedly an hereditary component in the transmission of diabetes; second, since 90 per cent of children developing diabetes have nobody in the immediate family with the disorder, the

---

Table 1. WHO classification of diabetes

A Clinical classes

Insulin-dependent diabetes mellitus (IDD)

Non-insulin-dependent diabetes mellitus (NIDD)
  Non-obese
  Obese

Malnutrition-related diabetes mellitus (MRDM)

Other types of diabetes associated with certain conditions and syndromes
  Pancreatic disease
  Disease of hormonal aetiology
  Drug-induced or chemical-induced conditions
  Abnormalities of insulin or its receptors
  Certain genetic syndromes
  Miscellaneous

Impaired glucose tolerance (IGT)
  Non-obese
  Obese
  Associated with certain conditions and syndromes

Gestational diabetes mellitus (GDM)

B Statistical risk classes (subjects with normal glucose tolerance but substantially increased risk of developing diabetes)
  Previous abnormality of glucose tolerance
  Potential abnormality of glucose tolerance

---

hereditary factor cannot be the only factor and is probably not the most important. Present evidence indicates that it is unlikely that the hereditary disposition to diabetes is due to a single recessive gene, but rather that varying combinations of alleles are responsible.

Histocompatibility antigens

The study of genetically determined antigens present on the surface of leucocytes called Human Leucocyte Antigens (HLA) has revealed an association between some of these antigens and various disease states. In particular, 90 per cent of insulin-dependent patients show either HLA DR3 or DR4 or both together and there is even closer association with DQB; DR2 appears to protect against disease. There is also an association with complement and other genes. Of course, this is not to say that all insulin-dependent diabetics have these particular haplotypes, but rather that individuals with this particular genetic make-up are more liable to develop diabetes.

Immunological factors

Antibodies to islet cell tissue have been demonstrated in newly diagnosed juvenile diabetics. Unlike antibodies formed in primary disorders of the immunity system, these antibodies are not persistent and gradually disappear. The role of these antibodies is still uncertain.

Environmental factors

Circumstantial evidence has accumulated which points to viral infection as the factor most likely to precipitate diabetes. Diabetes in children occurs very much less frequently in the summer than it does in the winter months, when virus infections are epidemic. Diabetes is known to occur following mumps; also babies born to mothers who have had rubella during preganancy are prone to develop diabetes. Children who develop diabetes have a higher incidence of antibodies to viral infections than non-diabetic children. Post-mortem material from children who have died shortly after the development of diabetes shows the islets to be infiltrated with lymphocytes and plasma cells very suggestive of a viral infection or immunological reaction. Animals inoculated experimentally with certain viruses have developed diabetes. All this evidence is very suggestive but so far definitive proof is lacking. If a viral infection is responsible, then one of at least two possibilities has to be explored. First, the infection may be nonspecific and diabetes results from the cumulative effects of several different viral assaults on the islets; or

second, the damage may be due to a specific virus, at present not yet identified or even known, as was the case with hepatitis.

The explanation of the aetiology of juvenile-onset type diabetes must encompass all the factors discussed. The most likely hypothesis is that the inheritance of particular haplotypes renders the islets susceptible to viral infections. The islets respond to the viral antigen by the production of antibodies. Cellular destruction ensues and this leads to the development of diabetes. It can be seen that many problems remain to be solved.

Type II diabetes (non-insulin dependent)

This is certainly the commonest type of diabetes, occurring most frequently in middle age but often in old age and occasionally in young adults. The diagnosis is often made by routine examination of the urine for sugar and the symptoms only elicited on direct questioning. Thirst, polyuria and loss of weight may be present but are seldom severe. In women, pruritus vulvae is often the presenting symptom. The diagnosis can be established by finding an elevated blood sugar or by performing a glucose tolerance test, if there is any doubt. The urine contains sugar but acetone is not found. Studies on plasma insulin show that insulin is present, but usually at levels lower than normal.

Inheritance

Unlike type I diabetes, there is no preponderance of particular HLA haplotypes. Although there is no doubt that maturity-onset diabetes occurs in families, two particular factors make it difficult to assess the type of inheritance. First, the diagnosis is often not specific and is based on the glucose tolerance test. Glucose tolerance deteriorates with age, however, so the dividing line between normal and abnormal is blurred. Second, this type of diabetes may not manifest itself until late in life and there is no certain way of detecting a predisposition to diabetes.

Occasionally, type II diabetes occurs in children or growing adults and in some families of this sort the inheritance may be dominant. When diabetes occurs in an identical twin, it is always concordant (both twins have diabetes) in the maturity-onset type, again suggesting a strong genetic inheritance.

Obesity

The nature of the inherited defect has not yet been elucidated but current evidence suggests that the islet cells are unable to respond completely to the stimulus of a raised blood glucose, perhaps due to

Table 2. Primary diabetes

	TYPE I	TYPE II
Common age of onset:	Any, predominantly young	Any, predominantly middle and older ages
Family history of diabetes:	Uncommon	Common
Seasonal incidence of onset:	More in winter months	No seasonal preponderance
Phenotype:	Thin	Obese
Haplotypes:	HLA B8, B15, B18, DR3, DR4, DQB, etc	No preponderance
Onset:	Rapid	Slow
Symptoms:	Severe	Mild or absent
Urine:	Sugar and acetone	Sugar
Keto-acidosis:	Prone	Resistant
Serum insulin:	Low or absent	Usually depressed but may be raised
Islet cell antibodies:	Present at onset	Absent
Treatment:	Insulin	Diet

an impoverishment of receptors on the islet cell surface. The factor most likely to precipitate the onset of diabetes in those who inherit this weakness is obesity. Overeating, particularly of carbohydrate foods, leads to increased demands for insulin and obesity causes resistance in the peripheral tissues to the action of insulin. It is well established that obesity is more common in type II diabetes than in controls. In families prone to diabetes, the disorder appears most frequently in those who are overweight.

In the light of these findings, the treatment of maturity-onset diabetes is self evident. The weight must be reduced, preferably by restriction of refined carbohydrates and saturated fats. This leads to an increased sensitivity to circulating plasma insulin and a return of blood sugar to normal in most cases. In some cases, despite dieting, the blood sugar remains elevated and in these, oral hypoglycaemic agents may be prescribed. The sulphonylureas lead to an increased output of insulin from the beta cells.

Although there are distinct aetiological, pathogenetic and clinical differences between insulin-dependent and non-insulin-dependent diabetes, similarities also exist. Both types of diabetes may occur in the same family, though this may be no more than might be expected by chance. Certainly, both types may develop the same degenerative changes in the blood vessels, nerves, kidneys and eyes, suggesting therefore that the degeneration is due to hyperglycaemia rather than to any inherited aetiological factor. Further, although in the initial stages the maturity-onset diabetic may have a nearly adequate insulin supply, this may ultimately fail and insulin may be necessary therapeutically.

Diabetes associated with other genetic disorders

Diabetes is sometimes a part of somewhat rare syndromes occurring in childhood and involving the neuro-endocrine and nervous system. Perhaps the least uncommon is the DIDMOAD syndrome. DIDMOAD is an acronym for diabetes insipidus, diabetes mellitus, optic atrophy and deafness. (Friedreich's ataxia, polyneuritis, retinitis pigmentosa, hypogonadism and obesity are other features sometimes involved.) The genetic inheritance of these disorders can hardly be in question because they often occur in siblings or when the parents are consanguinous. The most likely explanation is that the syndrome is due to an inherited defect of embryonic neuroectoderm, from which primitive endocrine cells migrate to the gut and pancreas. There are many other associations with genetic disorders.

Secondary diabetes

Diabetes results from destruction of the islets by surgery, disease or drugs.

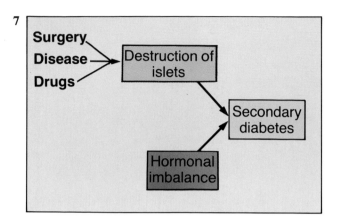

7   Secondary diabetes: aetiology known.

Surgery

At least three-quarters of the pancreas can be removed without diabetes resulting, providing that the remnant is healthy. Because the pancreas is the sole source of insulin, diabetes inevitably follows total pancreatectomy.

Disease

Acute pancreatitis can cause diabetes, which is often temporary.

Chronic pancreatitis, especially when associated with alcoholism, leads to progressive destruction of both exocrine and endocrine cells and eventually diabetes ensues. Calcification in the pancreatic area may be seen on Xray and a retrograde pancreatography reveals a dilated duct. Calcific pancreatitis associated with diabetes is more often seen in tropical countries and in some parts of South Africa and Southern India.

Haemochromatosis is an inherited disorder in which excess iron is absorbed and deposited in various organs including the liver, heart, pancreas and testis. Fibrosis of the tissues results, leading to cirrhosis and to diabetes. Nevertheless, deposition of iron causing fibrosis of the pancreas does not appear to be the only factor. The incidence of diabetes in haemochromatosis is considerably higher in cases with a family history of diabetes, suggesting an hereditary tendency must also be present for clinical diabetes to ensue. When diabetes is associated either with firm hepatomegaly or with a subtle grey skin pigmentation, the diagnosis of haemochromatosis must always be considered. The diagnosis can be confirmed by the findings of a high serum iron, a low total iron binding capacity and a high iron saturation. A liver biopsy reveals gross deposition of iron in the hepatic parenchyma and bile duct epithelium, distinguishing the condition from haemosiderosis.

Carcinoma of the pancreas may lead to diabetes, often without extensive destruction of the pancreas by the growth, perhaps because the growth stimulates destruction of the remainder of the pancreas by antigenic action. Diabetes is more likely to occur with growths in the tail of the pancreas, because this is the main site of the islet cells and further extension to the head may lead to jaundice as well. Diabetes appearing in an elderly patient associated with loss of weight and abdominal or back pain must always give rise to fears of carcinoma, particularly if jaundice occurs.

Drugs

Apart from hormones (discussed later) the benzothiazide diuretics can frequently exert a diabetogenic effect, probably by suppressing islet cell release of insulin. Diazoxide, at first used in the treatment of hypertension, is the most powerful diabetogenic agent of this group and can be used in the treatment of hypoglycaemia induced by islet cell tumours. Streptozotocin is another agent which has a direct destructive action on the beta cells, though its main application is in inducing diabetes in experimental animals: its only clinical use is occasionally in the treatment of hypoglycaemia due to an insulinoma. Alloxan is another powerful suppressant of the beta cells but its use is confined to experimental animals.

Hormonal imbalance

The action of insulin is unique in that it is the only hormone which can reduce the level of sugar in the blood. Several hormones are capable of increasing the level of sugar in the blood, mainly by increasing the formation of glucose in the liver (gluconeogenesis) or by converting hepatic glycogen to glucose (glycogenolysis). If these hormones are produced or given in excess, secondary diabetes may occur, usually subsiding when the hormonal stress is removed.

Cortisone

Cortisone increases hepatic gluconeogenesis and blocks the peripheral utilisation of glucose, so that about a third of patients with Cushing's syndrome have an elevated blood glucose. The clinical presentation of diabetes associated with plethora and hypertension should always arouse suspicion of Cushing's syndrome.

Cortisone, when given for therapeutic reasons, may lead to temporary diabetes, particularly when the dose is large or is maintained over long periods, as is sometimes necessary in asthma, systemic lupus or in association with immunosuppressive drugs. Patients on steroid therapy should be monitored for glycosuria and hyperglycaemia.

Growth hormone

This has a diabetogenic action by stimulating lipolysis and mobilising glycerol, thus opposing the peripheral action of insulin. Hypophysectomy performed leads to vastly increased sensitivity to insulin. Experimentally, repeated injections of growth hormone can cause diabetes in animals.

From the clinical viewpoint, about a quarter of patients with acromegaly develop diabetes, particularly those with a family history of this disorder.

Glucagon

This is produced by the alpha cells of the islets and has an action opposite to that of insulin. It converts liver glycogen to glucose and can be used therapeutically in the treatment of hypoglycaemic attacks induced by excess insulin. It promotes lipolysis.

In insulin-dependent diabetes, glucagon levels are often higher than normal and this may play a part in promoting hyperglycaemia and ketosis.

Tumours of the alpha cells (glucagonoma) lead to mild diabetes, loss of weight, stomatitis and a skin rash (migratory necrolytic erythema).

Adrenalin

Another hormone which mobilises glucose from hepatic glycogen is adrenalin. When produced in excess by a tumour of the adrenal medulla (phaeochromocytoma), diabetes may co-exist with hypertension. Unlike the hypertension, the diabetes is seldom severe. Both disorders remit following successful removal of the tumour.

Thyroxine

This increases intestinal absorption of glucose and promotes hepatic gluconeogenesis. It seldom causes diabetes, although in thyrotoxicosis glucose tolerance may be depressed and temporary glycosuria may appear.

Oestrogens

These are present in the contraceptive pill and may decrease glucose tolerance. The dangers of this aspect of contraceptive therapy have been exaggerated, especially with the introduction of low-dosage oestrogen tablets. There is no evidence to indicate that the pill causes diabetes and even in diabetics needing insulin, introduction of the pill does not usually lead to a significant increase of insulin dosage. Hormone replacement therapy (HRT) has no obvious effect on the control of diabetes.

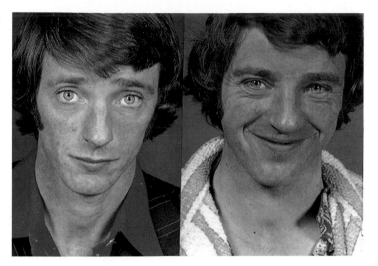

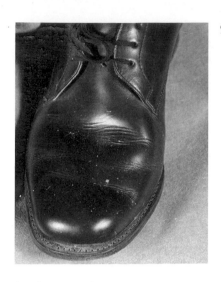

8 Newly diagnosed diabetic before and after only one week of insulin therapy.

9 Symptomless maturity-onset diabetes with sugar deposits on shoes from splashes of urine.

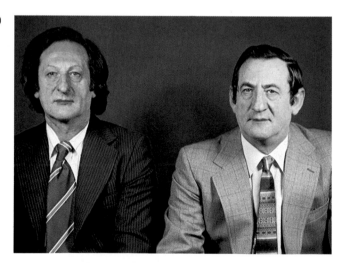

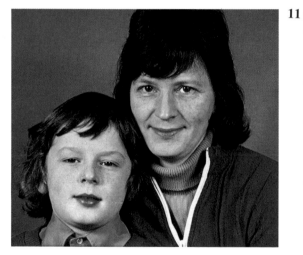

10 Type II diabetes (non-insulin-dependent) in identical twins. Both developed the disorder in their early 50s. Diabetes is nearly always concordant in identical twins with non-insulin-dependent diabetes. In identical twins, one of whom develops insulin-dependent diabetes, the other twin has no more than a 30 per cent chance of developing diabetes.

11 Type I (insulin-dependent). Mother and child both on insulin, an unusual occurrence. Only 10 per cent of newly diagnosed children have a first-degree relative with diabetes.

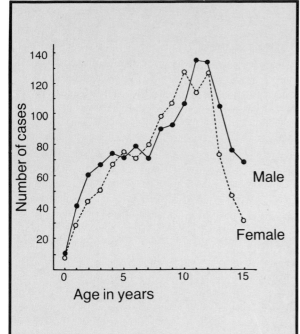

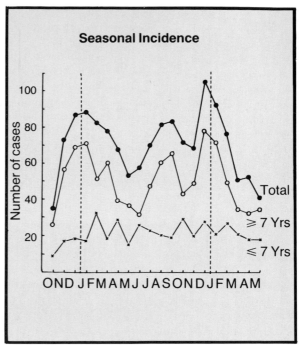

12 Incidence of diabetes in newly diagnosed children, showing peak at 11-12 years of age.

13 Seasonal incidence of diabetic onset showing that nearly three times as many of the older children develop the disorder in the winter months, suggestive evidence of a viral infection.

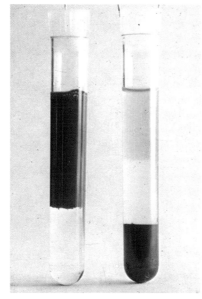

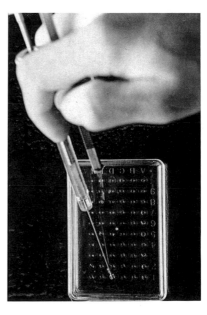

14 Histocompatibility antigens (HLA) in diabetics. Method of identifying the antigens on the surface of human leucocytes. On the left, a sample of defibrinated venous blood layered on to a separation medium and on the right, after centrifugation, the clear leucocyte layer lying above the red cells.

15 Dispensing leucocyte layer on to a microtest plate containing wells of different HLA antisera.

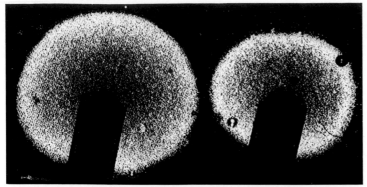

16 Leucocyte migration technique (LMT). On the left leucocytes have migrated normally from the capillary tube into the culture medium. On the right migration has been inhibited by the presence of pancreatic antigen, indicating that there is altered cellular immunity in diabetes.

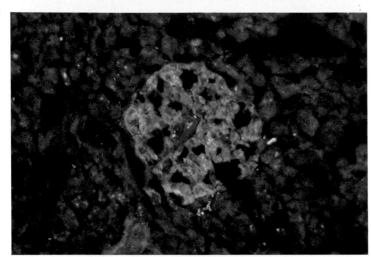

17 Pancreatic islet cell antibodies in diabetes demonstrated by fluorescent technique. Cryostat section of human pancreas treated with serum from a diabetic patient showing fluorescence in all islet cell types. (× *400*)

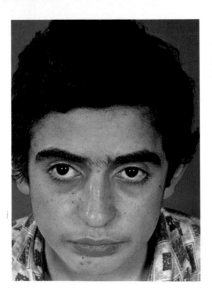

18 Diabetes insipidus, diabetes mellitus, optic atrophy and deafness (DIDMOAD), probably due to a genetic defect of the neuro-endocrine system.

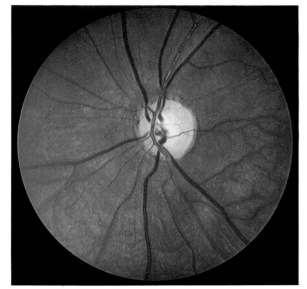

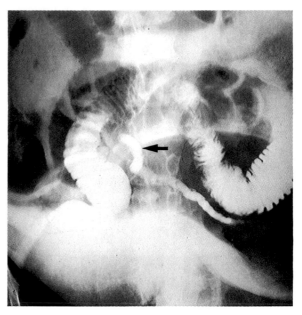

19 Retina showing optic atrophy in DIDMOAD. Blindness and diabetes in this syndrome are both determined genetically.

20 Endoscopic retrograde cholangio-pancreatography (ERCP) demonstrating dilated pancreatic duct in chronic pancreatitis (arrowed).

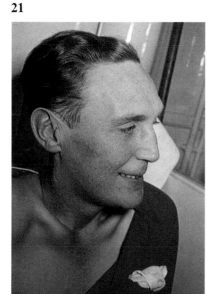

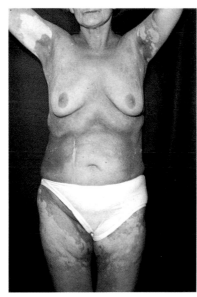

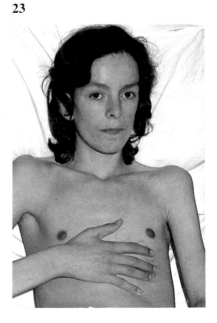

21 Haemochromatosis. Characteristic skin pigmentation which has led to the alternative description 'bronzed diabetes'.

22 Autoimmune disease. Diabetes mellitus and vitiligo. Other autoimmune disorders such as pernicious anaemia, Addison's disease and hypothyroidism may also co-exist.

23 Autoimmune disease. Diabetes mellitus and Addison's disease, both diagnosed simultaneously. Pigmentation on fingers. Antibodies present to islet cells and adrenals.

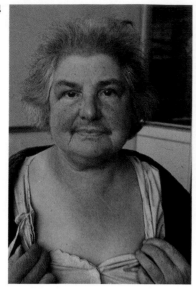

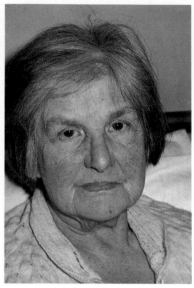

24   Diabetes, hypertension and plethora: basophil adenoma of pituitary: Cushing's syndrome.

25   Normal blood glucose and blood pressure in same patient (**24**) following pituitary ablation.

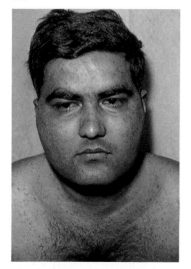

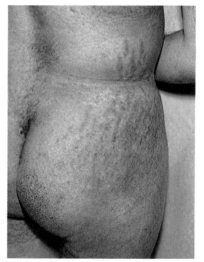

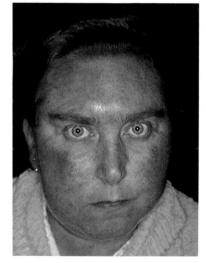

26   Cushing's syndrome due to adrenal hyperplasia, no evidence of pituitary adenoma. High plasma ACTH and cortisol values besides glucose intolerance.

27   Cushing's syndrome showing striae (same patient as **26**). This patient was cured by bilateral adrenalectomy but may later develop a pituitary adenoma (Nelson's syndrome).

28   Cushing's syndrome due to adrenal adenoma. Low plasma ACTH, high plasma cortisol and impaired glucose tolerance. Treated by removal of adrenal tumour.

29

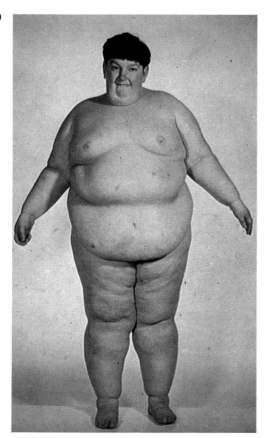

29 Prader-Willi syndrome. Diabetes is often present. Gross obesity, small genitalia and small hands are common.

30

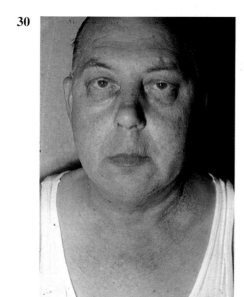

30 Carcinoma of the bronchus presenting as diabetes mellitus. High plasma ACTH and cortisol values, with hypokalaemic alkalosis.

31

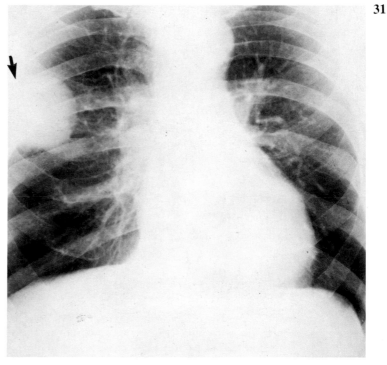

31 Carcinoma of the bronchus (arrowed) seen on chest Xray.

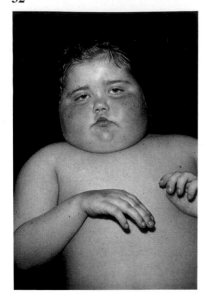

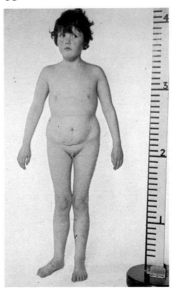

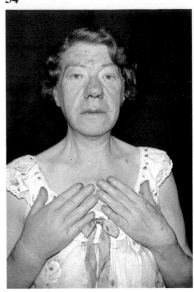

32 Child with nephrotic syndrome treated by steroids in large doses. Developed diabetes requiring insulin while on steroid therapy.

33 Normal glucose tolerance in the same child 3 years later with complete recovery on discontinuation of steroids.

34 Diabetes and acromegaly: 50 per cent of acromegalics develop glucose intolerance at some stage, although only half of these go on to frank diabetes and few require insulin. Those with a family history of diabetes are more prone to develop diabetes.

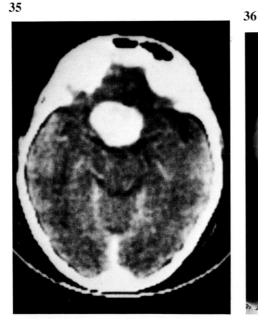

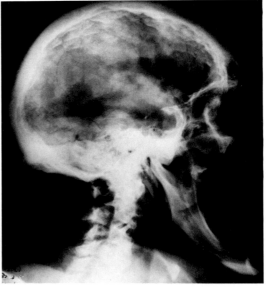

35 Pituitary adenoma. Computerised tomographic (CT) scan showing horizontal slice above the level of the pituitary after IV injection of vascular contrast agent. Dense white sphere (arrowed) confirms a large supracellar extension of a pituitary adenoma.

36 Acromegalic skull with secondary diabetes. Hypertrophy of the cranium, significant enlargement of the jaw and large pituitary fossa.

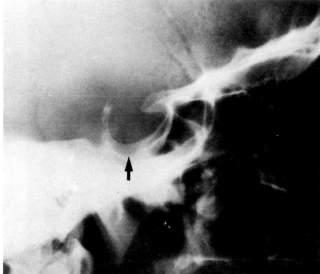

37 **Pituitary fossa** in detail showing typical 'ballooned' enlargement of the fossa with double floor (arrowed) due to a pituitary adenoma.

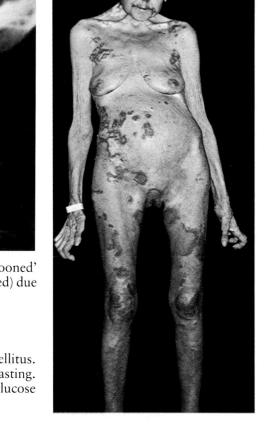

38 **Glucagonoma** with mild diabetes mellitus. Migratory necrolytic erythema and muscle wasting. Glucagon secreting tumour removed and glucose tolerance restored to normal.

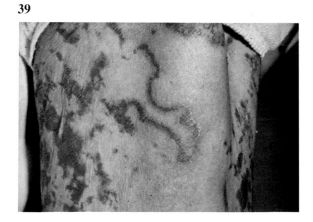

39 **Necrolytic erythematous rash** in detail from picture **38.**

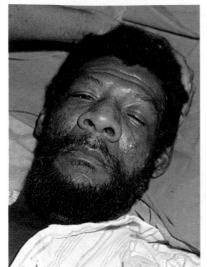

40 Phaeochromocytoma presenting with hypertension and diabetes mellitus. Although most cases have impaired glucose tolerance, only about 10 per cent have overt diabetes.

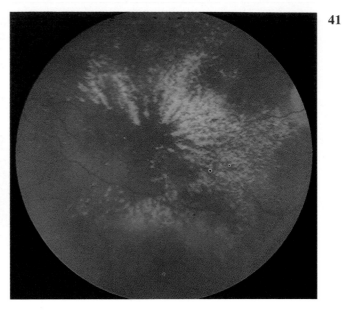

41 Fundus (from **40**) showing macular star of hypertensive retinopathy.

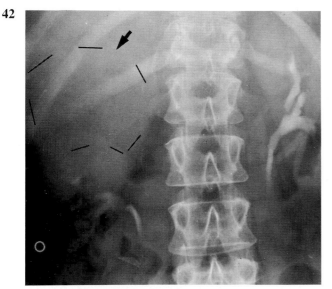

42 Phaeochromocytoma IVP showing depressions of right kidney by large suprarenal mass (arrowed).

43 Suprarenal mass (arrowed) above right kidney revealed by arteriogram in capillary phase. This large phaeochromocytoma was successfully removed with restoration to normal of blood pressure and blood glucose.

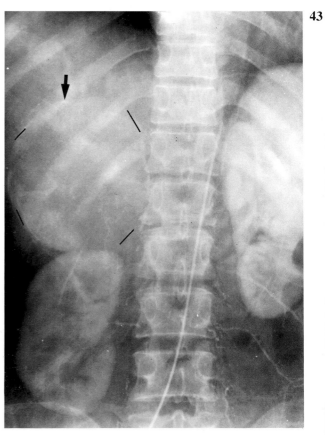

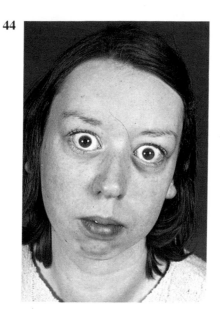

44 Thyrotoxicosis with temporary glycosuria and hyperglycaemia.

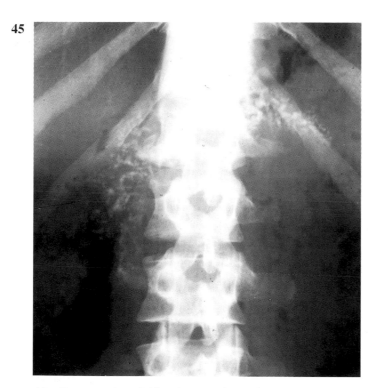

45 Pancreatic calcification resulting from pancreatitis.

3 The pancreas

Study of the pancreas in man has been hindered by the difficulty in obtaining biopsy tissue. In animals, destruction of islet tissues with alloxan or streptozotocin to create the metabolic environment of diabetes inevitably distorts observation of the islets' response in idiopathic diabetes. Nor are studies of the intact pancreas in animals entirely relevant to the human types of the disorder.

The normal pancreas varies in weight between 60g and 160g. About 3 per cent of the total is composed of islet tissue which tends to be more evident in the tail. There is a wide variation in the number of islets, the average being about 1 000 000. Islets also vary in size: in obese individuals and in the infants of diabetic mothers, gross hypertrophy of the islets may be seen with islets of 400µm in diameter. Approximately 80 per cent of cells are the insulin producing beta (B) cells, 15 per cent are glucagon secreting alpha (A) cells, while the remainder are either delta (D) cells producing somatostatin or PP cells producing pancreatic peptide.

Whereas the purpose of the D cells has not been fully elucidated they do not, as was previously believed, secrete gastrin. They are now known to secrete the tetradecapeptide somatostatin, which is also produced by the hypothalamus. The hormone has a profound inhibitory effect upon the secretion of insulin and glucagon. Other cells have been identified which produce pancreatic peptide (PP), a hormone which probably exerts a regulatory effect upon glucose homeostasis in response to feeding.

Nerve fibres have been detected which lie between the exocrine and islet tissue and have been shown to secrete vasoactive intestinal polypeptide (VIP). This hormone can stimulate production of insulin, although its relationship to diabetes mellitus remains speculative.

Insulin synthesis within the beta-cell cytoplasm first involves the formation of pre-proinsulin under the influence of messenger-RNA. Ribosomes transfer RNA amino acids to make the A, B and C chains of proinsulin (see **46**). The chains, linked in the order A-C-B, are formed close to the microsomal membrane. The pre-hormone sequence is cleaved away so that folded proinsulin with its A,B and C chains can be identified in the endoplasmic reticulum. Secretion granules containing the A and B chains of insulin separated from the connecting C peptide appear in the region of the Golgi zones of the beta-cell cytoplasm, ultimately to be secreted from the cell by emiocytosis.

Alpha cells can generally be distinguished by their elongated nuclei and by granules more closely concentrated and of greater density than those of the beta cells. In insulin-dependent diabetes the chief lesions found in the islet tissue of the pancreas are: hyaline change; fibrosis; and lymphocytic infiltration ('insulitis'), loss of B cells and sometimes fibrosis, leaving A and B cells intact. In non-insulin-dependent diabetes, amyloid deposition in the islets can be striking and may replace B cells. It consists of islet amyloid polypeptide (IAPP), but its precise role is still disputed. It is not specific for diabetes.

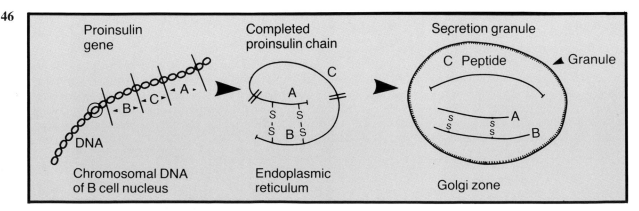

46

Proinsulin gene

Completed proinsulin chain

Secretion granule

C Peptide ▲ Granule

C

A

s s

s B s

Chromosomal DNA of B cell nucleus

DNA

A

s s

B

s s

Endoplasmic reticulum

s s A

s s B

Golgi zone

46 Insulin synthesis within the beta-cell cytoplasm.

Lymphocytic infiltration ('insulitis')

This lesion has been most commonly reported in the younger patient coming to post-mortem within a short time of the onset of severe diabetes. In its most advanced form the whole pancreas may be red and swollen with marked infiltration of the islets by lymphocytes and large mononuclear cells. All islet-cell types may be infiltrated and destroyed, although in milder cases there may be mixed fibrosis and predominant destruction of beta cells. With the ability to measure islet-cell antibodies (ICA) in the serum of juvenile-onset diabetics, this lesion has acquired greater significance. The fact that ICA are most commonly found only as a transient phenomenon coincident with the onset of type I diabetes (see Chapter 2) and that lymphocytic infiltration occurs in similar circumstances, suggest that both represent the effects of an antigen-antibody reaction causing islet-cell destruction.

Other pancreatic lesions

Fibrosis

Fibrosis of the exocrine pancreas, both interlobular and interacinar, is perhaps the simplest and commonest lesion in the pancreas.

Lipomatosis

Fatty infiltration of the pancreas as a whole correlates closely with the fat distribution of the patient and thus is most marked in obese diabetics.

Vascular disease

Although arteriosclerosis of pancreatic vessels may be marked, especially in the elderly, it is less than that of the spleen which shares the same vascular circuit; thus vascular disease is unlikely to be a significant cause of diabetes even in the elderly.

Pancreatitis

Acute haemorrhagic pancreatitis with fat necrosis is often associated with transitory hyperglycaemia. The combination of acute pancreatitis with severe diabetic metabolic decompensation is unusual and carries a poor prognosis. Chronic pancreatitis, especially when associated with stone formation which predisposes to fibrosis and islet loss, is more commonly associated with diabetes mellitus. Overall 20-40 per cent of cases having chronic pancreatitis develop glucose intolerance; so this diagnosis must be considered when the onset of diabetes is associated with episodes of epigastric pain.

Carcinoma of the pancreas

Diabetes is most commonly a consequence of carcinoma of the head of the pancreas, despite the fact that most of the islets are in the tail. When diabetes and jaundice develop within a few weeks of each other, the diagnosis is nearly always carcinoma of the pancreas.

Insulinoma

Clinically, insulin secreting tumours are the most important cause of hypoglycaemia in the non-diabetic. Although 85 per cent of lesions are benign, it is not possible to distinguish clinically whether a tumour is benign or malignant. Indeed, only those lesions which metastasise can confidently be regarded as malignant. Most insulinomas are between 1cm and 2cm in diameter, but may be as small as 0.5mm or as large as 15cm. Because resection can dramatically cure the presenting symptoms, careful localisation of the abnormal tumour circulation by angiography is invaluable, if surgery is to be undertaken. Rare ectopic lesions can similarly be demonstrated pre-operatively.

Insulinoma can also occur in diabetics although with no greater frequency than in the general population. Immunoassay of the C-peptide of proinsulin has greatly facilitated diagnosis in the diabetic routinely treated with exogenous insulin, because the level of C-peptide is a measure of endogenous insulin production.

Multiple micro-adenomata of the pancreas may be derived from B cells and so be insulin secreting; or they may be composed of gastrin-producing cells giving rise to the Zollinger-Ellison syndrome characterised by gastric hypersecretion, ulcer formation and diarrhoea.

Glucagonoma

Tumours of the glucagon-secreting alpha cells lead to mild diabetes mellitus. The diagnosis should be considered when glycosuria is associated with the skin rash of migratory necrolytic erythema, weight loss and stomatitis. Patients are ill, and the prognosis poor.

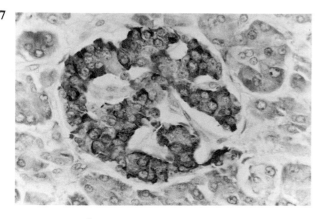

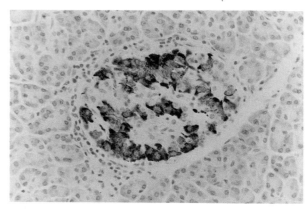

47 Beta cells in a normal islet (*Immunoperoxidase* (I.P.) for insulin × 500).

48 Early insulitis. There is relatively little loss of beta cells and there is a peripheral infiltrate of small lymphocytes. I.P. for insulin.

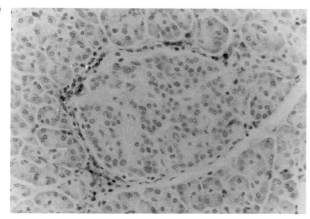

49 I.P. for leucocyte common antigen (× 350).

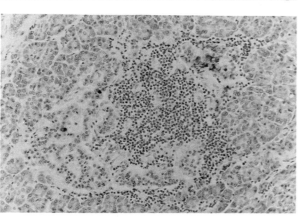

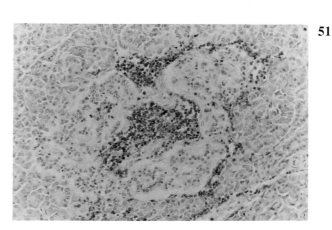

50 Advanced insulitis. There is a marked reduction in the number of beta cells accompanied by a diffuse infiltrate of lymphocytes. I.P. for insulin.

51 I.P. for leucocyte common antigen (× 220).

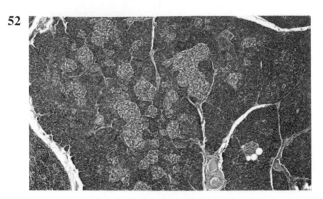

52 **Islet-cell hyperplasia** in obese diabetic. Section of pancreas showing an increased number of islets in the field.(*H&E × 30*)

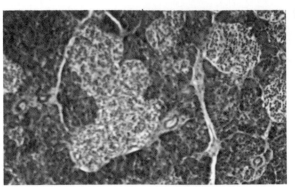

53 **Enlarged islet** magnified from **51.** (*H&E × 80*)

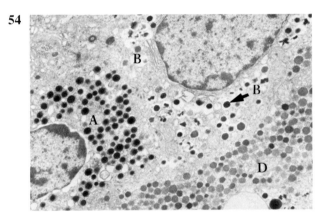

54 **Islet cell** showing alpha (A), beta (B) and delta (D) cells. Electron micrograph at ultrastructural level. (× 6 000)

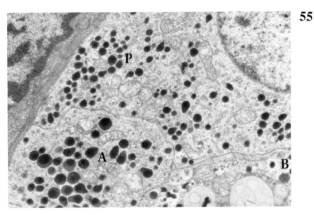

55 **Alpha (A), beta (B) and pancreatic peptide (P) cells** in detail from similar electron micrograph. (× 10 000)

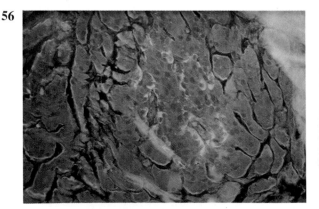

56 **Human pancreatic islet** with antibodies to glucagon to demonstrate the presence of the hormone in the A cells. (*Immunoperoxidase × 400*)

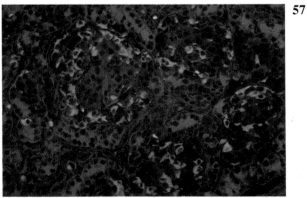

57 **Human pancreas using antibodies** to somatostatin to demonstrate the hormone in the D cells. (*Immunoperoxidase × 400*)

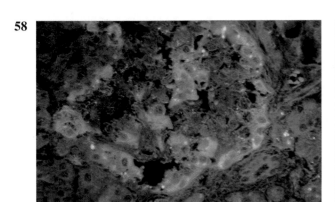

58 Antibodies to pancreatic polypeptide (PP) showing the hormone in the PP cells. (*Immunoperoxidase* × *400*)

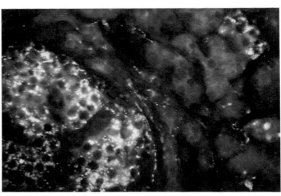

59 Human pancreas stained with antibodies to vasoactive intestinal polypeptide (VIP). VIP is a neurotransmitter found in the thread-like nerve fibres seen here surrounding the islet. VIP causes release of insulin, although its rôle in the pathogenesis of diabetes is unknown. (× *400*)

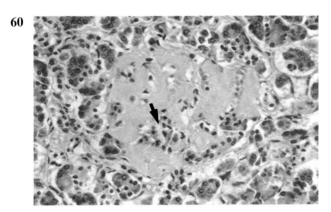

60 Amyloid of the pancreatic islet. Pink amyloid tissue containing remnants of islet cells (arrowed). (*H&E* × *300*)

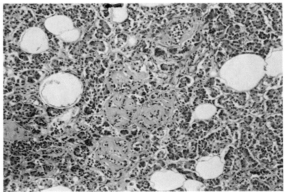

61 Focal fatty change and hyalinised islets. Scattered fat vacuoles with pink hyaline material within the islets. (*H&E* × *80*)

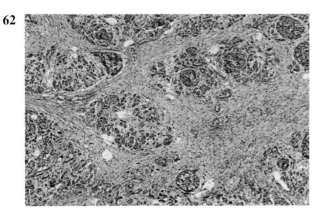

62 Pancreatic fibrosis showing a widespread fibrous reaction in the interstitial tissue. (*H&E* × *30*)

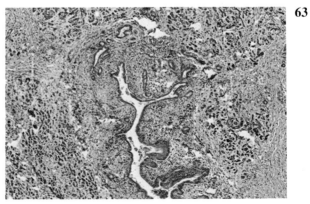

63 Pancreatic fibrosis showing periductal fibrous reaction. (*H&E* × *30*)

64

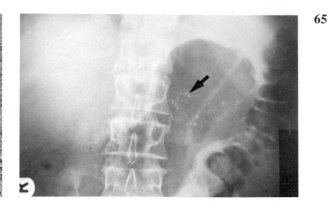

64 Pancreatic fibrosis showing a widespread fibrous reaction in the interstitial tissue, but leaving the islets (arrowed) essentially intact. (*H&E × 30*)

65

65 Chronic pancreatitis with calcification. Plain Xray film of abdomen showing stippled calcification (arrowed) in pancreas seen through a large gastric air bubble.

66

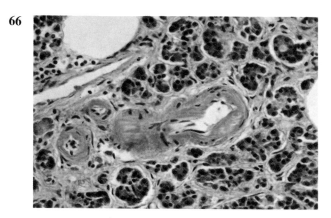

66 Hyalinised arteriole in pancreas. Elderly hypertensive diabetic with widespread arteriolar disease at autopsy. (*H&E × 300*)

67

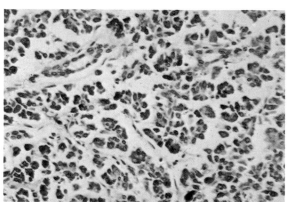

67 Haemochromatosis showing blue staining iron in the exocrine pancreas. (*Perl × 150*)

68

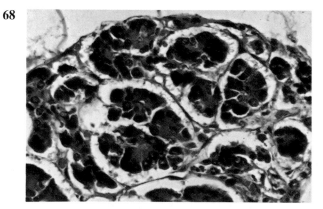

68 Haemochromatosis showing iron deposition in pancreatic tissue. (*H&E × 400*)

69

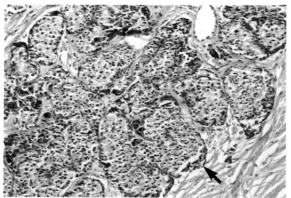

69 Islet-cell adenoma showing the lobulated pattern (arrowed) of proliferating islet cells. (*H&E × 80*)

70 **Islet-cell carcinoma** showing a diffuse pleomorphic pattern with loss of the usual islet-cell architecture. (*H&E × 80*)

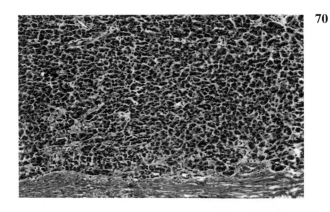

71 **Poorly differentiated adenocarcinoma of pancreas** with small area of normal pancreatic tissue in upper right hand corner of section. (*H&E × 30*)

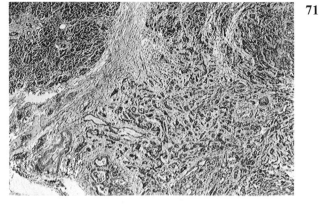

72 **Normal islet from the glucagon rich lobe of the pancreas** stained by an immunoperoxidase technique for insulin (× 160).

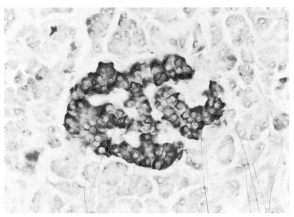

73 **A similarly stained islet from a child who died in ketoacidosis** at presentation of acute onset diabetes. Note the striking reduction in the number of insulin-containing cells. Many other islets were completely depleted of insulin (× 160).

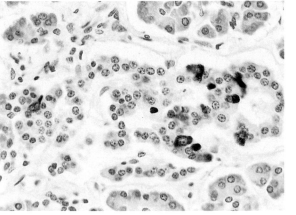

74

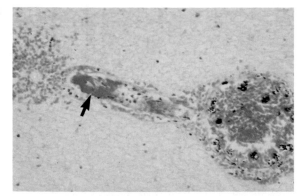

74 Disseminated intravascular coagulation. Section of brain from a patient who died in ketoacidosis showing a vessel with a side branch containing fibrin and distally a small petechial haemorrhage (arrowed).(× 400).

75

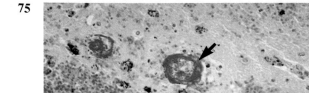

75 Disseminated intravascular coagulation. Section of brain showing two blood vessels containing fibrin (arrowed) stained red with Martius-Scarlet-blue stain. (× 400)

76

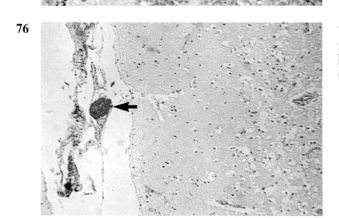

76 Meningeal vessel containing a clump of red fibrin (arrowed) in section of brain. Marked vacuolation of neurones and glial cells of cerebral cortex. (*MSB* × 400)

4 The liver

Although diabetes mellitus involves a marked disturbance of intermediary metabolism, the liver, which is the organ chiefly concerned in the metabolism of carbohydrate, shows little upset in its other biochemical functions. Nor is the liver affected by the serious long-term complications of diabetes which damage the nervous system, large blood vessels, the small vessels of the kidney or the retina.

In newly diagnosed or poorly controlled diabetes the liver is often enlarged and soft. Histological examination shows fatty infiltration, which regresses as the diabetes comes under control with treatment.

A large firm liver on clinical examination suggests the possibility of diabetes secondary to haemochromatosis or hepatic infiltration associated with pancreatic neoplasia. Although diabetes has little serious adverse effect upon the liver, hepatic disease may cause secondary diabetes. Glycogen storage disease leads to hepatomegaly in children and may cause glucose intolerance. The relationship between the liver and diabetes can be complex. Patients having liver disease tend to show a marked hyperglycaemia following meals, and yet on fasting, the hepatic ability to release glycogen is impaired.

Hence, there may be swings from post-prandial hyperglycaemia to fasting hypoglycaemia. The relationship may be further complicated by impaired insulin breakdown by the liver. This favours hypoglycaemia and causes altered carbohydrate or lipid metabolism in peripheral tissue. This, in turn, enhances glucagon secretion and so restores hyperglycaemia.

The liver is involved in two important metabolic pathways affected by diabetes mellitus: gluconeogenesis and fat synthesis.

Gluconeogenesis

In severe insulin lack, the liver is supplied with massive amounts of free fatty acids (FFA). These are oxidised in the liver, simultaneously releasing large quantities of ketone bodies into the circulation. At the same time release of amino acids from breakdown of protein or lactate production in peripheral tissue supplies the liver with the carbon substrates essential for glucose formation. This process, which can be a useful source of both glucose and ketone bodies for energy in times of starvation, accelerates hyperglycaemia and keto-

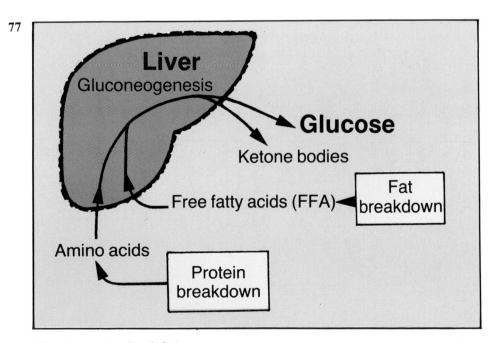

77   Severe insulin deficiency.

acidosis in the severe insulin deficiency of insulin-dependent diabetes. Moreover, the hormones of stress—cortisol, catecholamines, glucagon and growth hormone—may individually or collectively antagonise the action of insulin during intercurrent illness. Subsequent lipolysis from peripheral fat stores may burden the liver with a massive supply of free fatty acids to fuel the gluconeogenic process. Not only does the consequent hyperglycaemia exceed the renal threshold for glucose, so opening the flood gates of an osmotic diuresis, but the output of ketone bodies by the liver far exceeds the needs of muscle or other tissues. Thus ketone bodies (3-hydroxybutyrate, aceto-acetate and acetone) swamp the circulation with organic acids leading to acidosis and acidaemia. The latter induces rapid (Kussmaul) breathing and since acetone is volatile, this causes the characteristic smell in the patient's breath.

Insulin is the essential hormone in arresting gluconeogenesis. Its most immediate effect is to restrain fatty acid release from adipose tissue (the antilipolytic effect). By reducing the supply of FFA, the energy source for hepatic gluconeogenesis is removed. Subsequently, the presence of insulin in the liver antagonises the key enzymes of gluconeogenesis.

Fat synthesis

Whereas gluconeogenesis characterises the insulin deficient diabetic, the pathway followed by fatty acids in the liver of the obese or mild maturity-onset diabetic is mainly in the direction of triglyceride synthesis. Excess carbohydrate consumption in the obese untreated diabetic favours hepatic triglyceride synthesis. Alcohol, cortisol or any underlying liver disease will all stimulate this pathway. The triglyceride is released into the circulation as very low-density lipoprotein (VLDL) or pre-beta lipoprotein. Although triglyceride predominates, cholesterol will also be synthesised in the liver in similar circumstances. Both forms of lipid synthesis account for the fatty liver of the untreated obese diabetic. When there is underlying liver disease (or excess alcohol consumption), the transfer of triglyceride and cholesterol into pre-beta lipoprotein is impaired. In such instances fatty infiltration of the liver is most marked and soft hepatomegaly most easily detected clinically.

Although the fatty liver is characteristic of the mild obese diabetic, similar changes can be induced in poorly controlled insulin-dependent patients, especially when diet adherence is poor and calorie intake excessive. The insulin-dependent diabetic may also develop glycogen infiltration in circumstances of chronic insulin overdosage. Excess insulin will stimulate the pathways of glycogen storage. It follows that erratic patients who swing between poor control and insulin excess may show, on liver biopsy, a mixed picture of fatty infiltration and glycogen storage.

78   Mild diabetes: residual insulin action.

79 Fatty liver. Section showing diffuse vacuolation of hepatocytes, a common finding in newly diagnosed or poorly controlled diabetics. (*H&E × 200*)

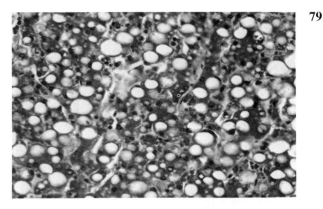

79

80 Glycogen-laden liver cells. Section shows clear plant-like pattern, sometimes found in diabetics chronically overtreated with insulin. (*H&E × 200*)

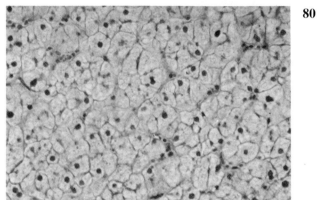

80

81 Hacmochromatosis. Section of liver showing blue-stained iron deposition in liver cells and fibrous connective tissue. (*Prussian blue × 30*)

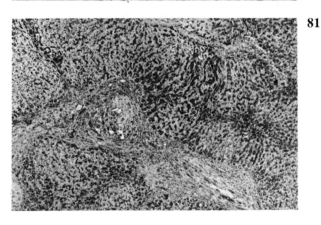

81

82 Haemochromatosis. Detail of liver cells showing iron deposition. (*Prussian blue × 200*)

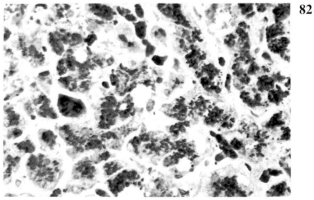

82

83

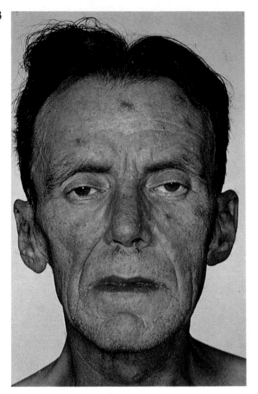

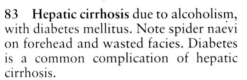

84

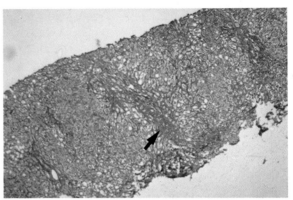

83 Hepatic cirrhosis due to alcoholism, with diabetes mellitus. Note spider naevi on forehead and wasted facies. Diabetes is a common complication of hepatic cirrhosis.

84 Fibrous tissue (arrowed) and regeneration of liver cells typical of alcoholic cirrhosis. Section of liver biopsy from patient in **83**. (× 25)

5 Management

The management of diabetes depends very much on the proper education of those who develop the disorder so that they can look after themselves intelligently. They must fully understand the aims of treatment and how to achieve them. There is no use expecting diabetics to follow rules and restrictions unless they appreciate the purpose of the advice given to them. This is as true for elderly non-insulin-dependent diabetics as it is for children needing insulin.

Modern education will entail not only personal instruction and explanation by the physician, the nurse and the dietitian but also group instruction, parent-child meetings and educational holidays. Instructional pamphlets, books, tapes and videos are all valuable in helping the diabetic to help himself.

Diet: healthy eating

Diet plays an integral role in the control of diabetes and yet every survey shows that most diabetics in practice do not accurately follow dietary instruction. The reasons for failure of compliance are at least threefold. First, not enough time is spent on explaining the purpose of the diet and what can be achieved. Second, the diet recommended is too remote from the habits, customs and capabilities of the diabetic concerned. Third, the diet sheet is too detailed and complicated for the uninitiated to follow.

Hence, it is important to explain carefully the aims of the diet, to find out what the diabetic normally eats and to alter it as little as possible. Thus, the diabetic should be provided either with a simple diet sheet that can be understood and followed or be given a demonstration of healthy foodstuffs, using specially prepared visual displays. The diet must be individualised according to the age, background and intelligence of the patient.

In non-insulin-dependent diabetes, the total calorie intake of the diet at onset will depend on the weight of the patient. The greater the degree of obesity, the greater the restriction on the calorie content of the diet. About half the energy content of the diet should be carbohydrate and the mainstay should be complex carbohydrate with integral fibre: refined carbohydrates, particularly sugar, should be avoided. Thus, wholemeal bread, wholewheat pasta, wholegrain breakfast cereal, brown rice, vegetables (especially beans and pulses) and fresh fruit are to be encouraged while sugar, jams, cakes, chocolates, sweet drinks and biscuits should be avoided.

Total fat consumption should be reduced and polyunsaturated fats should replace saturated animal fats. This means that fried foods, potato crisps, chips, butter, cream, sausages, hamburgers and meat fat should not be encouraged. Butter can

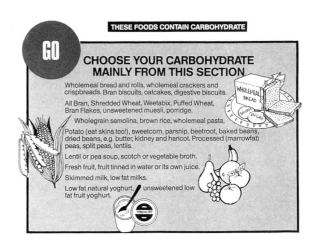

85 and **86** **Dietary advice.** Diet sheets are now replaced by booklets and other aids aimed at better understanding by the patient.

be replaced by polyunsaturated vegetable fat or low fat substitutes. Skimmed milk can replace rich milk. Cottage cheese can replace high fat cheese.

Protein is provided by poultry, lean meat and fish. Milk, cheese and eggs are also valuable sources of protein and for vegetarians, peas and beans will make up any deficit.

Even when oral hypoglycaemic agents are prescribed, the timing of meals in this type of diabetes is not crucial.

In diabetics needing insulin, the food recommendations remain the same, but stress is now on making sure that an adequate amount of food is eaten commensurate with the activity, age, weight and appetite of the patient. If the patient is thin or underweight, the diet must be sufficient to restore the weight that was lost at the onset of diabetes. The meals must now be spaced at regular intervals in order to prevent hypoglycaemia. These are, usually three main meals (breakfast, lunch and dinner) often with snacks mid-morning, mid-afternoon and at bed-time, according to the type of insulin and when the injections are given.

Once the principles of the diet are understood, there is no need for food to be dull or repetitive and the term 'diet' can be replaced by 'healthy eating'.

Exercise

Exercise is crucial in diabetes, because physical activity assists in reducing blood glucose levels, as well as being helpful in combating obesity and hypertension. Clearly, the type of exercise recommended has to be monitored in the light of the patient's age, weight, previous activity, general health and inclination. For the elderly with a tendency to obesity, walking and swimming can be recommended. For the more energetic, a skipping rope, static bicycle and rowing machine offer opportunity for more vigorous exercise in the home.

For the young diabetic taking insulin, exercise should be part of the general approach to good health and keeping fit. Vigorous exercise enhances absorption of subcutaneously injected insulin and increases utilisation of blood glucose, both factors leading to the dangers of hypoglycaemia. This should never be considered a bar to sporting activities. It is is important to remember that extra refined carbohydrates such as biscuits or a sandwich should be taken before a game of squash or jogging, and glucose or dextrose sweets should be readily available on the person and taken during exercise. Many celebrated athletes on insulin have learned how to avoid hypoglycaemia while pursuing their sport in this way.

Oral hypoglycaemic agents

Oral hypoglycaemic agents are used in the treatment of patients with non-insulin-dependent diabetes who have failed to respond to dietary restriction and exercise. If despite improved eating habits and an increase in physical effort, random blood glucose levels remain elevated, say above 10 mmol (180 mg/dl), then tablets can be used.

Two types of tablets with different modes of action may be prescribed. The first is metformin, a biguanide. Metformin is a mild hypoglycaemic agent, probably acting by delaying absorption of monosaccharides from the bowel and by reducing the output of glucose from the liver into the blood. It reduces serum cholesterol. Metformin gives rise to some nausea and diarrhoea but, perhaps because of its anorectic effect, usually leads to a reduction in weight which is especially desirable in the obese diabetic. Consequently, metformin may be the first choice in an overweight diabetic who has failed to respond to advice on diet and exercise.

The sulphonylureas are the most widely prescribed oral hypoglycaemic agents and, if properly used, have been shown to be safe, well tolerated and, within limits, effective in reducing the blood sugar levels. They act primarily by stimulating the beta cells of the pancreas to produce more insulin and so are ineffective in insulin-dependent diabetics where the pancreas is incapable of producing insulin. Once again it should be stressed that these tablets should only be introduced when an adequate trial of diet and exercise have failed to reduce the blood glucose to a satisfactory level.

There are many types of sulphonylurea tablets now available and all have the same range of effect. However, some have a short duration of action and should be taken two or three times a day, while others have a longer effect and need be taken only in the morning before breakfast. The dose prescribed will depend on the response of the blood glucose: once normoglycaemia is achieved, the dose should be progressively reduced to the minimum effective dose necessary to maintain suitable blood glucose levels. In some cases, the tablets can be discontinued if normoglycaemia can now be maintained on diet alone.

On the other hand, if the maximum dose of the sulphonylurea prescribed is ineffective, metformin can be added. If this too does not restore near normoglycaemia, then insulin therapy should be considered promptly.

The introduction of a sulphonylurea often leads to an increase in weight, partly because of the restoration to normoglycaemia and better metabolic control. Remember that many drugs (for example MAO inhibitors, sulphonamides, salicylates and phenylbutazone) enhance the hypoglycaemic effect of the sulphonylureas. Many patients previously well controlled on tablets show temporary loss of control in the face of infection. It may be necessary to institute insulin until the infection has been overcome and often tablet therapy can then be re-introduced in place of insulin.

Insulin

Insulin is necessary to preserve health in non-keto-acidotic diabetics who fail to respond adequately to diet and tablet therapy, and to sustain life and preserve health in insulin-dependent diabetics who usually present in ketoacidosis or who are prone to develop ketoacidosis under the stress of infection or other illness (see **Table 3**).

Source

Insulin is available from animal sources (beef and pork) and from genetically manipulated bacterial sources. Purification of insulin has progressed steadily since the first crude preparation in 1922 and its antigenic propensities have steadily diminished. It is now rare to see gross fat atrophy or distressing local allergy at the site of injection and unusual to find, as often was the case, insulin resistance requiring hundreds of units of insulin daily. Insulin extracted from porcine sources is slightly less antigenic than that from beef. Human insulin is now generally available, derived from two sources, one as a derivation of porcine insulin and the other as a genetic manipulation of the plasmid of *E.coli*, which then provides the components for constitution into human insulin. Thus, for the first time, insulin is available from non-animal sources. In practice, very little difference can be found between purified pork or human insulin.

Duration of action

There are various types of insulin preparations. Neutral soluble insulin is quickly absorbed but the effect lasts only a few hours. Hence, modifications have been prepared by which the absorption and effective action can be prolonged. For example, isophane insulin is a suspension of insulin with protamine which prolongs effective action to about 8 hours.

Amorphous insulin zinc suspension has a similar length of action. By crystallising insulin and using a zinc suspension, the activity of a single injection is further prolonged to about a day. Consequently, the various preparations of insulin can be described as short, intermediate and prolonged. There are several preparations of fixed mixtures of short and intermediate action but many diabetics prefer to individualise by mixing soluble and isophane themselves in their syringes.

Table 3. Commonest available insulins in the UK

Soluble insulins	Mixtures
Human Actrapid©*	Human Initard© (50% velosulin, 50% insulatard)
Humulin S©†	Human Mixtard© (30% velosulin, 70% insulatard)
Human Velosulin©* (also porcine)	(also porcine Mixtard and Initard)
	Human Actraphane© (30% actrapid, 70% protaphane)
	Humulin M1© (10% humulin S, 90% humulin I)
Isophane insulins	Humulin M2© (20% humulin S, 80% humulin I)
Human Insulatard©* (also porcine)	Humulin M3© (30% humulin S, 70% humulin I)
Humulin I©†	Humulin M4© (40% humulin S, 60% humulin I)
Human Protaphane©*	
Zinc suspensions	
Humulin Lente©†	
Humulin Zn©†	
Human Monotard©*	
Human Ultratard©*	

* Enzymatically manipulated pork (emp).
† Biosynthetic human insulin (prb).
Bovine insulins are still available as Hypurin Neutral©, Isophane©, Lente© and Protamine Zinc© from CP Pharmaceuticals. Other insulins such as Rapitard©, Lentard© and Semitard© are still available.

Administration

Disposable plastic syringes with attached needle are now used by most diabetics. They are sterile before use and can safely be used for at least five injections, after which the needle tends to get blunt. Pen syringes are also available and rapidly gaining in popularity (see below). In the UK, USA, Canada and Australia the insulin is 100 units per ml strength, whereas in some parts of Europe the insulin is still 40 or 80 units per ml strength. Consequently, it is important to check markings on the syringe to make sure that they correspond to the strength of insulin used.

There are various routines available for the administration of insulin. Many diabetics who have failed to respond to tablets, and elderly patients, can manage quite satisfactorily on a single morning injection of an intermediate or long-acting insulin. Most young and active insulin-dependent diabetics need insulin twice daily or more frequently. For example, a fixed mixture of short and intermediate insulin administered 40 minutes before breakfast ensures good control for the morning and afternoon and a further injection before the evening meal covers the evening and overnight. Most diabetics require about 60 per cent of the total dose before breakfast and 40 per cent before the evening meal.

For those diabetics not well controlled on this simple routine, it may be necessary to give a long-acting insulin (perhaps 40 per cent of the total requirement as basal therapy) before bed-time and bolus doses (perhaps 20 per cent of the total) before breakfast, lunch and the evening meal. Pen syringes are now available, can be carried on the person and contain the insulin necessary for the bolus dose before each meal. The insulin is contained in a cartridge and a system of clicks or a dial denotes the dose of insulin administered. This is not only particularly useful for those diabetics with impaired vision, but also makes injecting convenient and more accurate for those with busy daily routines.

Continuous subcutaneous insulin infusion (CSII)

A further refinement of insulin administration is provided by a portable infusion pump. This administers continuous insulin via a plastic tube connected to a butterfly needle inserted under the skin usually, of the abdominal wall.

There are several suitable infusion pumps, mostly delivering insulin from a reservoir syringe. The pump is carried in a holster and as well as ensuring a steady basal flow of insulin day and night, allows a bolus dose of insulin to be administered 30 minutes before each main meal.

The portable pump has provided excellent control of diabetes in many diabetics previously unhappy with their regime. It demands understanding and self-discipline on behalf of the diabetic and the back-up of a diabetic centre experienced in this field and adequately staffed to cope with difficulties and emergencies. Patients are usually admitted to the centre for a few days for instruction and institution of this therapy. They are taught how and where to insert the subcutaneous needle, how to refill the reservoir of insulin, how to administer the pre-meal booster dose and how to disconnect the pump temporarily for purposes such as a bath.

Among the hazards of this form of therapy is the fortuitous interruption of insulin delivery due to disconnection of the tube from the needle, failure of the battery, kinking of the tube or clogging of the needle. Since there is no reservoir of insulin subcutaneously, ketoacidosis can occur within a few hours. Many diabetics feel the pump an encumbrance to wear, time consuming to set up and find the site of the subcutaneous cannula may be sore or even become infected. Hence, although the pump suits a few diabetics, it certainly does not suit all; there is an increasing preference for techniques using pen syringes.

Hypoglycaemia

Hypoglycaemia can be induced by insulin-producing tumours, by the sulphonylureas by various drugs (including alcohol) and, most commonly, by insulin administered in treatment. Since cerebral tissue needs a constant supply of glucose for its metabolism, even temporary deprivation leads to perceptible changes in cerebral function and ultimately to coma. If hypoglycaemic coma is allowed to persist too long, irretrievable cerebral damage occurs.

The symptoms of insulin-induced hypoglycaemia (see **Table 4**) are conditioned by the rate at which the blood glucose falls and the depth to which it falls. A rapid fall in blood glucose due to an excessive amount of insulin leads to an adrenalin response with symptoms of sweating, anxiety, restlessness, tremor, hunger, circumoral paraesthesia and palpitations. Later, there are symptoms of cerebral dysfunction with slurred speech, double vision, inco-ordination, confusion and loss of insight. Either situation can lead to coma unless it is treated. Very rarely decerebration or death can ensue if the hypoglycaemic state is allowed to persist for many hours, although particularly in young people, spontaneous recovery is more likely to occur.

Loss of warning of hypoglycaemia is a common problem, and as a result every insulin-dependent diabetic must be aware of the dangers of hypoglycaemic reactions and how to avoid them. Education of the newly diagnosed diabetic requiring insulin will include explanation of the time and duration of action of the insulin injections, the importance of spacing the meals and the role of exercise. Stress will be laid on the need to carry glucose sweets (or a convenient equivalent) always on the person and the advisability of taking action at the first symptom of hypoglycaemia, usually easily recognisable by the diabetic himself, though often idiosyncratic. The spouse or parent of a child with diabetes should also be instructed what to look for and what to do. When on holiday and medical help is not easily available, a glucagon kit may be invaluable. 1 mg glucagon can be injected subcutaneously or intra-muscularly if the diabetic is unable to take glucose by mouth, and when recovery occurs, usually in about 20 minutes, a warm glucose drink followed by food can then be given.

Oral hypoglycaemic agents, particularly the sulphonylureas, can lead to hypoglycaemia especially if their action is augmented by other drugs. For example, phenylbutazone, salicylates, anti-depressants, MAOI and some anticoagulants can enhance the hypoglycaemic effect of the sulphonylureas. Hypoglycaemia induced in this way has a gradual onset and responds to intravenous dextrose; glucagon can be given as well, because this mobilises hepatic reserves of glucose from glycogen (see Table 5).

Table 4. Symptoms and signs of hypoglycaemia

Early warning	Shaking, trembling
	Sweating
	Pins and needles in tongue and lips
	Palpitation
	Hunger
	Headache (especially early morning)
Neuroglycopenia	
Mild	Double vision
	Difficulty in concentration
	Slurring of speech
	Withdrawal/silence
Moderate	Confusion
	Change in behaviour
	Truculence
	Misbehaviour in children
	Restlessness with sweating
Late	Epileptic fits, especially children
	Hemiplegia in elderly (rare and reversible)
	Unconsciousness

Table 5. Suitable treatment for hypoglycaemia

Lucozade	60ml (2 fl oz)
Ribena	15ml (0.5 fl oz)
Coca-cola (not Diet)	80ml (3 fl oz)
Sugar	2 teaspoons
Sugar lumps	3 small
Dextrosol	3 tablets

Each item contains 10g of carbohydrate.

87

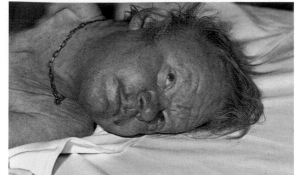

87 **Hypoglycaemia** induced by the maintenance of chlorpropamide therapy for diabetes and the introduction of monoamineoxidase inhibitor (MAO) therapy for depression. Some drugs (such as MAO inhibitors, sulphonamides, salicylates) may enhance the hypoglycaemic effect of oral agents. Treatment requires intravenous glucose and glucagon given subcutaneously or intramuscularly. Good recovery was achieved in this patient.

88

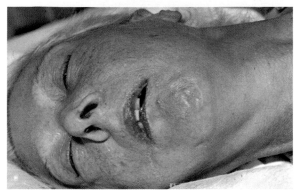

88 **Fatal hypoglycaemia** following irreversible cerebral changes. Insulin was self-administered by this diabetic woman with subsequent heavy intake of alcohol. She was left unattended for many hours before admission to hospital and failed to respond to glucagon and intravenous dextrose. Alcohol inhibits hepatic gluconeogenesis and so sustains hypoglycaemia.

89

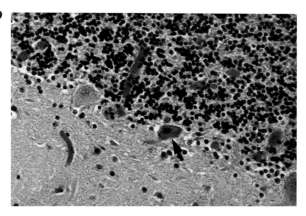

89 **Degeneration of Purkinje cells** with dense pyknotic nucleus (arrowed). Section of cerebral cortex from **92** ($\times$ *150*)

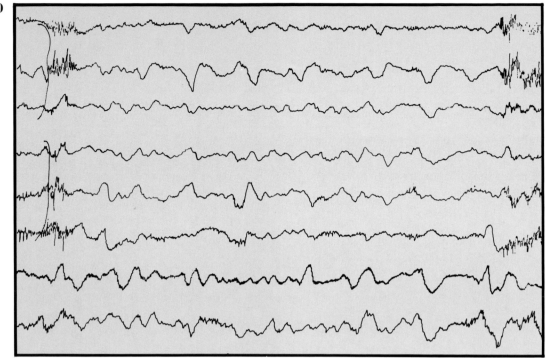

90 Suppression of alpha rhythm with generalised activity of slow delta waves. (*Electroencephalogram of patient in* **88**)

Diabetic ketoacidosis

Ketoacidosis occurs as a result of insulin deficiency. Blood ketone bodies (acetoacetate and 3-hydroxbutyrate, both acids, and acetone) increase to cause a metabolic acidosis, and blood glucose increases and leads to dehydration.

It is usually do to:

- Stopping insulin or reducing the dose, in error or deliberately;

- Resistance to insulin during infections;

- The unrecognised onset of insulin-dependent diabetes.

The clinical onset of ketoacidosis occurs over hours or days. Symptoms of uncontrolled diabetes are always present. Vomiting in insulin-dependent diabetes is always serious. The development of ketoacidosis is often unrecognised both by patients and doctors; it should be preventable by advice on insulin usage and the correct method of managing diabetes in the event of intercurrent illness.

The clinical features of ketoacidosis include severe dehydration associated with drowsiness (rarely unconsciousness); patients overbreathe and their breath smells of acetone (to those who can detect its scent). Many have gastric stasis and gastric splash. The more severe the cases are hypothermic and hypotensive. Aketotic cases are similar but without overbreathing or the smell of acetone.

91

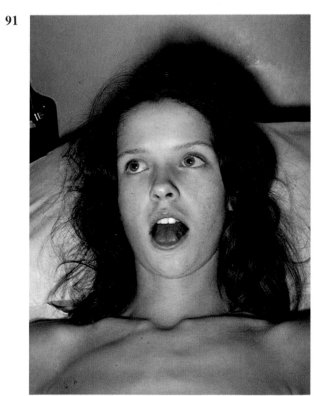

92

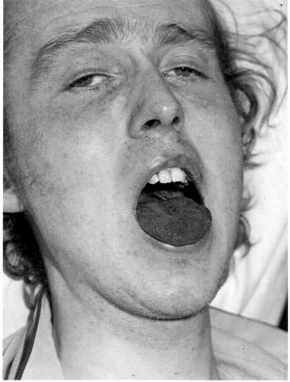

91 Ketoacidosis in a young girl; diabetes has been newly diagnosed.

92 Ketoacidotic pre-coma precipitated by omission of morning insulin injection because of nausea and vomiting.

Monitoring

Although there is probably a genetic component to the propensity to develop microvascular complications, there is strong experimental, clinical and epidemiological evidence that poorly controlled diabetes over the years contributes significantly to the evolution and progression of these complications. Hence, diabetics must be educated to monitor their response to treatment, so that therapy can be modified if the control is not satisfactory.

Urine testing

Whereas in most people, when the blood glucose exceeds about 8 mmol (144 mg/dl), glucose appears in the urine, this is by no means always so. The amount of glycosuria depends on the ability of the renal tubules to reabsorb glucose from the glomerular filtrate. In some cases (low renal threshold) glucose appears in the urine even when the blood glucose is within normal limits: in others, especially in elderly non-insulin-dependent diabetics, glucose does not appear in the urine even when the blood glucose exceeds 12 mmol (216 mg/dl)(high renal threshold); nor is the renal threshold necessarily always the same in the same patient. Consequently, at best the urinary glucose is a poor and inaccurate reflection of what is happening in the blood. Nevertheless, urine is readily available and offers some guide as to progress. It is most useful to test urine that has not been long in the bladder and passed before meals.

There are several simple tests available for assessing glycosuria depending on a change of colour of impregnated strips after dipping in the urine. Tes-Tape changes from yellow to green (1 minute). Clinistix© changes from pink to purple in 10 seconds when glycosuria is present, but the range of colour is limited. This test is useful only for screening but not for monitoring. Diastix© changes from green to brown (30 seconds). These tests are simple to perform and, providing the limitations are understood, yield helpful information.

Blood testing
(Home monitoring blood glucose)

Self-monitoring systems are now widely available for diabetics to test their own blood glucose levels.

These systems are valuable both in educating diabetics as to when, why and how their blood glucose levels fluctuate and also as a method of achieving better control by allowing intelligent adjustments of diet and insulin in response to blood glucose readings. Blood is obtained, usually from the pulp of a finger, either by applying a specially available lancet (monolet) into the finger or, preferably, by using a spring-loaded mechanical device. A blob of blood is now squeezed on to the reagent strip. Various reagent strips are available (for example, Dextrostix©, BM Glycemie, Visidex II or Hypoguard GA© test strips) and at the end of the specified time the blood is either washed off or wiped off, according to the strip used, and compared with the colour chart. Although the colour ranges are demarcated to give a reasonably accurate evaluation of the blood glucose, assessment is open to subjective bias. Particularly with children, there is a natural wish to choose the better figure where doubt exists. For this reason, many prefer the use of a meter which allows more objective evaluation of the blood. The strip is placed in the machine and by means of a photo-electric cell an accurate figure of the blood glucose appears on the screen. The most recent system, namely the ExacTech system, is much simpler to use, and the results obtained in just 30 seconds: no washing or wiping of blood is required. Because of its simplicity, it is probably more reliable. Its presentation as a pen makes it easy to carry in a pocket or handbag.

Glycosylated haemoglobin

Glycosylation of haemoglobin occurs gradually and consistently throughout the 120-day life span of the erythrocyte. In non-diabetics, about 6-8 per cent of haemoglobin (HbAl) is glycosylated but in poorly controlled diabetics the percentage may be 12 per cent or more. Hence, the degree of glycosylation is unaffected by temporary fluctuations in blood glucose levels and gives an overall picture of control. Conversely, it may take several weeks before improvement in control leads to a significant fall in glycosylation.

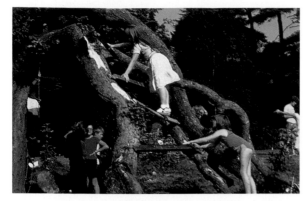

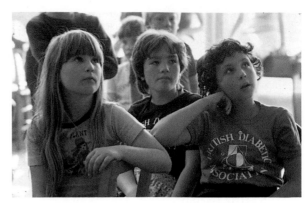

93 Educational holidays for children with diabetes.

94 Group instruction in general.

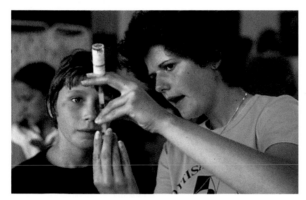

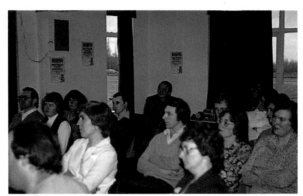

95 Individual explanation.

96 Lectures and discussion groups for parents of diabetic children.

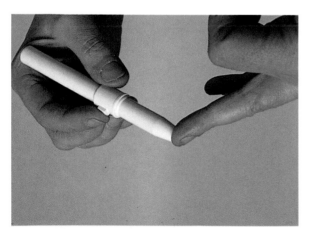

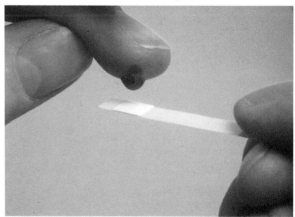

97 **Glucolar**© **pen** (soft touch).

98 **Blood glucose monitoring.** Applying drop of blood to dry biochemistry test strip.

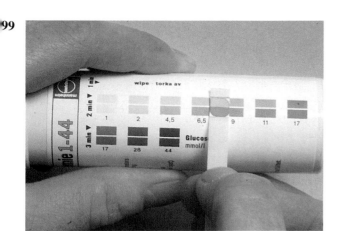

99 **Blood glucose monitoring.** After careful timing, visual reading of blood glucose value using colour scale.

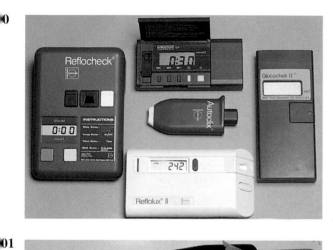

100 **Blood glucose monitoring.** Various battery-operated portable devices for measuring blood glucose.

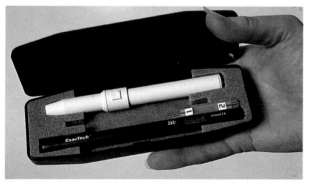

101 ExacTech© kit with calibration electrode.

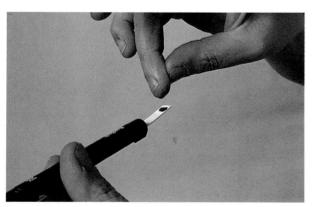

102 Blood sample on an ExacTech© pen.

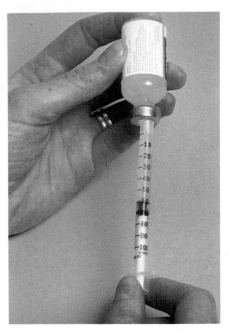

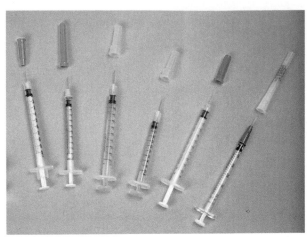

104   Plastic insulin syringes calibrated in units (100 units—1 ml).

103   Preparing insulin for injection.
Drawing insulin from vial into plastic syringe.

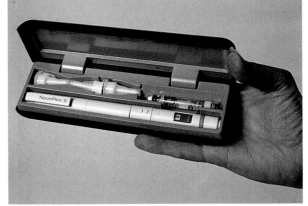

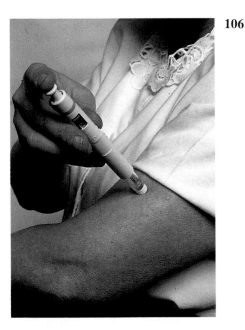

105   Novopen kit.

106   Novopen being used for injecting insulin.

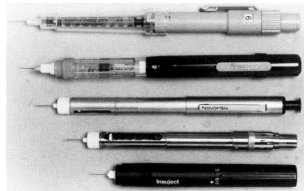

107 **Various pen syringes** for ease of insulin injecting.

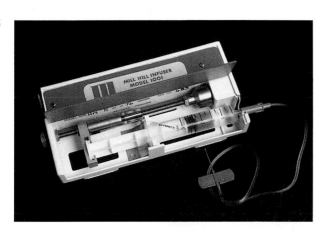

108 **Portable pump** for continuous subcutaneous insulin infusion. An early model showing the syringe of insulin, the syringe-driving mechanism and the plastic tube with a needle for subcutaneous insertion in the abdominal wall.

109

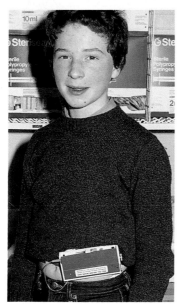

109 **Portable pump** for continuous subcutaneous insulin infusion (CS11). The newer range of pumps are even less bulky.

110

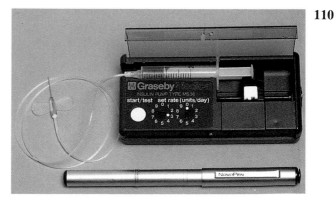

110 **Modern compact insulin infusion pump** alongside Novopen to demonstrate its size. Control dials for adjusting insulin infusion rate.

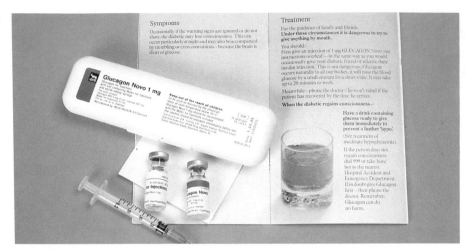

111 Pack of glucagon for hypoglycaemic emergencies. Glucagon in powder form is mixed with fluid and injected by the patient's relative or doctor using a sterile plastic insulin syringe.

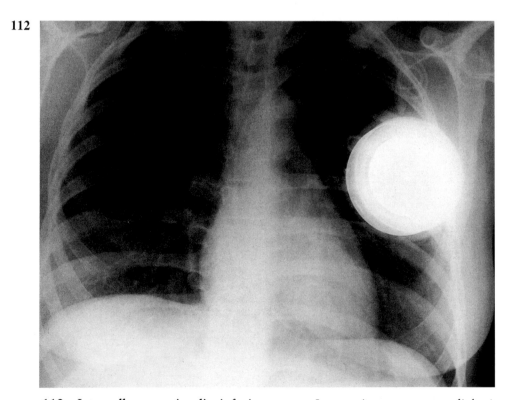

112 Internally worn insulin infusion pump. In rare instances some diabetic patients (usually female) are resistant to subcutaneous or intramuscular insulin. This constant speed pump is inserted in the pectoral region and the infusion line feeds into a suitable vein. The pump can be refilled through the overlying skin. Xray showing pump *in situ* and infusion line into vena cava.

6 Pregnancy, offspring and congenital malformations

The metabolic derangement that is present in the diabetic mother leads to changes in the growing fetus. Elevation of the maternal blood glucose is transmitted across the placenta and stimulates fetal insulin production with gross hypertrophy of the fetal islet cells, particularly after the 32nd week of pregnancy. Episodes of maternal ketoacidosis exert a deleterious effect on fetal metabolism. Indeed, poorly controlled diabetes in the mother is associated with a high fetal death rate. Apart from hyperglycaemia and ketosis, there is also evidence of hormonal imbalance in the diabetic pregnancy. Even when control of the diabetes is impeccable, the baby born to a diabetic mother is likely to be larger than average and Cushingoid in appearance. It is overweight, plethoric and fat. Respiratory distress syndrome (hyaline membrane disease) is now rare. The blood sugar at birth is often very low. Congenital abnormalities are more common in babies born to diabetic mothers, particularly such skeletal deformities as sacral agenesis and congenital heart disorders.

Three factors of management of the diabetic pregnancy have led to a significant improvement in the fetal loss rate of babies born to diabetic mothers, so that the fetal loss in well-run centres now hardly exceeds that occurring in the non-diabetic population.

Meticulous control of maternal diabetes before conception and throughout the pregnancy. This usually entails at least two injections of insulin a day, sometimes three or four. Self-monitoring of blood sugars by the patient is essential in maintaining them within the normal range. The diet must be nutritious, properly spaced and regular in time. Pre-conception counselling is always advisable.

Close co-operation between physician and obstetrician is necessary and the obstetrician must monitor the size of the fetus at regular intervals. The size of the fetus can be established by clinical examination and by ultrasound techniques. Interval ultrasonograms of the foetal head and girth help to assess the rate of growth in relation to dates. A large baby, particularly with obstetric complications such as a breech presentation, may suggest the need for a caesarian section at 38 weeks. Where the baby appears normal for size, and the pregnancy is uncomplicated, delivery at term is indicated by induction of labour, if required. The timing of delivery is of crucial importance. To induce too early means the delivery of a premature baby liable to death from respiratory failure. To wait too long increases the risks of intra-uterine death with an overlarge plethoric oedematous baby.

Care of the baby in a premature baby unit. The baby born of a diabetic mother sometimes though not always needs special care. The fetal blood sugar may be too low, so that dextrose should be administered. A good airway must be established. Oral feeding is usually established after 24 hours, and breast feeding is encouraged. When maternal lactation is satisfactory, breast milk can be expressed and fed to the baby until breast feeding is possible.

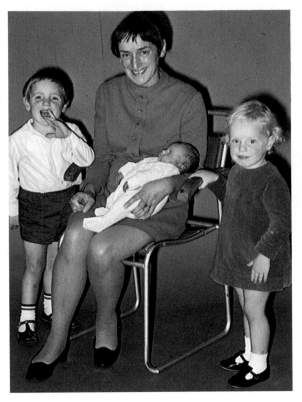

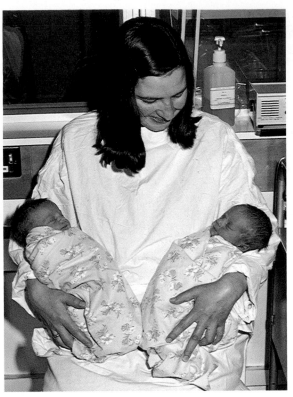

113 This woman had developed an insulin-dependent diabetes at the age of 18 years. She was well controlled on twice-daily insulin and enjoyed three successful pregnancies. In general more than two babies are not advised for a diabetic mother, because the burden of looking after the diabetes and a larger family may prove an undue strain.

114 A diabetic mother who was successfully delivered of identical twins via caesarian section at 38 weeks.

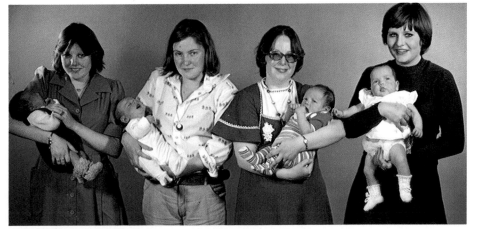

115 Four mothers with diabetes mellitus: all delivered healthy babies in the same week. The mother second on the left also has Addison's disease treated with cortisone. In well-organised centres, fetal mortality is now down to less than 2 per cent and is scarcely different from normal.

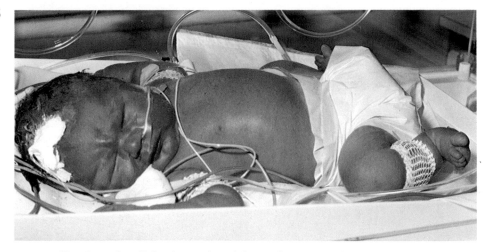

116 Offspring of a diabetic mother delivered at 38 weeks gestation. The infant is large, oedematous and plethoric. It received treatment at a premature-baby unit with satisfactory outcome.

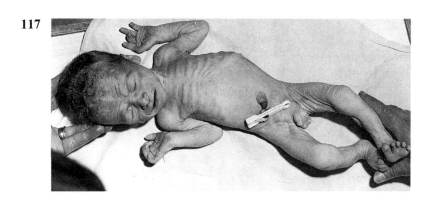

117 Transient diabetes mellitus is a very rare neonatal problem which should be suspected when grossly small-for-dates baby fails to gain weight despite having a voracious appetite. The infant is polyuric and glycosuric. Treatment with insulin is necessary. The condition remits spontaneously after a period of weeks or months. The aetiology remains unknown.

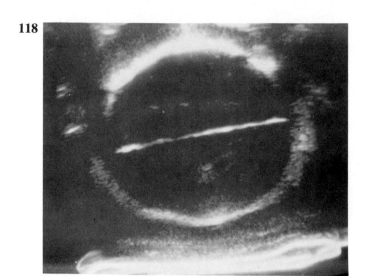

118 Biparietal cephalometry. Ultrasonogram showing mid-line foetal head at 33 weeks of diabetic pregnancy.

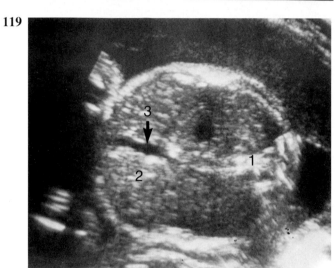

119 Fetal girth. These sonograms are a valuable indication of fetal size in relation to dates. (1 = spine, 2 = liver, 3 = umbilical vein).

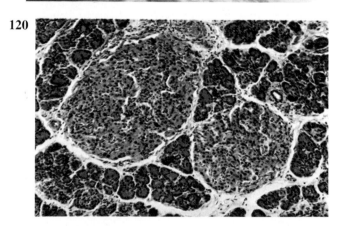

120 Gross hyperplasia of islet cells of pancreas in stillborn baby of diabetic mother poorly controlled and unsupervised during pregnancy. (× *150*)

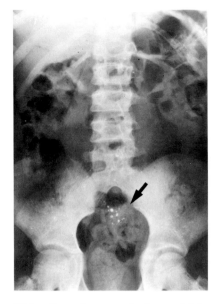

121 Sacral agenesis in a child.
The absence of the sacrum is a
rare congenital defect in the
general population which occurs
more frequently in the offspring
of diabetic mothers. (*Plain Xray*)

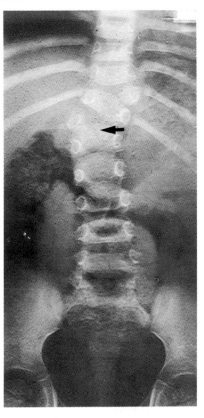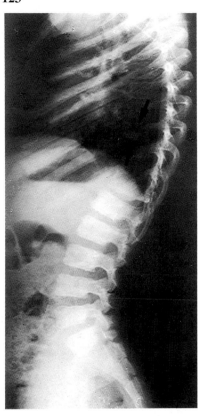

122 and **123   Vertebral agenesis** (arrowed) in a baby born to
a diabetic mother. (*PA and lateral Xrays*)

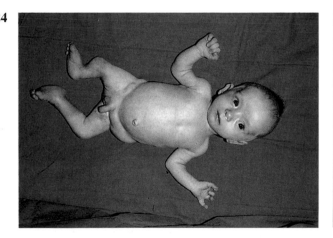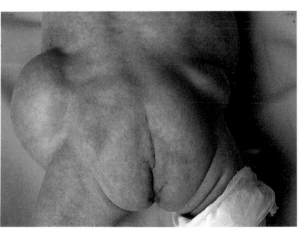

124 Male infant with inguinolumbar herniae,
lower limb deformities and undescended testes,
born to a diabetic mother.

125 Same infant as in 124 showing bilateral
herniae.

126

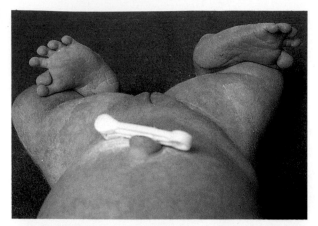

126 Female infant with left lumbar hernia and lower limb deformity.

127

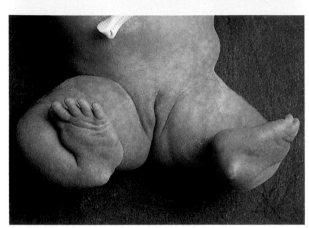

127 Same patient as in 126 showing absent tibiae, and polydactyly.

7 Peripheral vascular disease, neuropathy and the diabetic foot

Diabetics are liable to develop changes both in the large and small vessels. The term arteriosclerosis includes both atherosclerosis and medial calcification, although these two components may occur as separate entities. Microangiopathy refers to changes in the small vessels and capillaries and gives rise to ischaemic lesions in many systems, including the eyes, kidneys, skin and heart.

Atherosclerosis

This involves primarily the larger and medium-sized arteries and is characterised by fibrosis of the intima and the formation of subintimal fatty plaques. These plaques may calcify and ulcerate, providing a surface suitable for thrombus formation and consequent occlusion of the lumen. Although these pathological changes are not specific to diabetes, they occur at an earlier age in diabetics and tend to involve different vessels. In non-diabetics atherosclerosis is seen most prominently in the largest vessels, the aorta, the iliac vessels, the femorals and popliteals. In diabetics, it is the smaller vessels, particularly the tibials and popliteals, that are commonly involved.

Ischaemic heart disease

Coronary thrombosis has become the single commonest cause of death in diabetics. Moreover, a high proportion of non-diabetics suffering from myocardial infarction show an abnormal blood glucose response to oral glucose. The relationship between abnormal glucose metabolism, insulin and atheroma is complex. The chronic hyperglycaemia of uncontrolled diabetes leads to increased synthesis of mucopolysaccharides in the arterial wall and this favours the trapping of low-density lipoproteins. Thus, insulin lack is atherogenic, but increased circulating insulin actually stimulates the formation of atheroma in other ways. It inhibits the clearance of lipids away from the arterial wall and it provokes increased hepatic synthesis of plasma lipids. Many mild obese diabetics, or those treated with exogenous insulin, have excess of the hormone circulating from time to time—especially while fasting. Poorly controlled diabetics, with wide swings between hyperglycaemia and insulin-induced hypoglycaemia, may be the most vulnerable to atheroma. Diabetics tend also to have increased platelet adhesiveness and agglutinability, diminished fibrinolytic activity and increased blood viscosity at low and high shear rates, all of which are factors favouring intravascular thrombosis in those having atheroma.

The epidemiological risk factors for atheroma (obesity, hypertension and hypercholesterolaemia) are all more common in diabetics than in the general population. In whatever population group, whether of high or low prevalence of arterial disease, diabetes confers a twofold excess of clinical atherosclerosis. Moreover, the diabetic female loses the protection normally enjoyed by the non-diabetic female.

Despite the accelerated development of atheroma, the pathological changes in the vessels are not very different from those in non-diabetics. Diabetics tend to show a greater tendency to complicated lesions with plaque fissuring, rupture and ulceration. A greater area of vessel wall is involved and the atheromatous lesions extend into smaller arteries. Microvascular disease with thickening of the basement membrane of capillaries in the myocardium may either aggravate infarction or lead to ischaemic myocardial fibrosis, without either occlusion or other gross changes in the coronary arteries.

Peripheral vascular disease

Narrowing and occlusion of the arteries to the legs and feet often give rise to intermittent claudication on walking. Ischaemic pain may be present at rest with a sense of coldness in the affected limbs. Occlusion may occur suddenly, usually from thrombus formation in an already narrowed vessel, but sometimes from a dislocated atheromatous plaque and sometimes from an embolus formed in the heart. When this happens, pain in the affected limb may be severe and unremitting.

Examination of the legs for arterial insufficiency demands careful inspection of the skin, hair and nails. The skin over the feet and lower legs may be atrophic and hairless and the legs feel cold. The dorsalis pedis and posterior tibialis arteries in the feet and the popliteals and femorals in the legs should be identified. A bruit may be heard over the femorals, evidence of a significantly narrowed vessel. The use of Doppler ultrasound offers further guidance as to the severity of vascular disease but if vascular surgery or angiography are contemplated, arteriography is essential. Using the trans-femoral route, unequivocal information can be obtained as to the patency, size and regularity of the arterial tree from the origin of the common iliac to the foot pulses.

The feet

Diabetic foot problems result from either peripheral neuropathy associated with vigorous and intact vascular supply; or from the presence of peripheral vascular disease. When the two are present together, the ischaemia is the predominant or more serious problem. Care of the feet plays a crucial role in the prevention of disability. The diabetic often becomes divorced from his feet: poor vision prevents his seeing them and loss of sensation precludes his feeling them. Consequently, only a conscious programme of regular inspection and care can avoid unnecessary damage by trauma or heat. Trivial injuries in diabetics, if left unattended, can lead to adverse consequences for three reasons. First, ischaemia leads to impoverishment and devitalisation of the tissues, especially the skin. Second, neuropathy dulls sensation and allows trauma to persist unnoticed and without pain. Third, bacterial infection flourishes when the blood sugar is elevated and when the tissues are deprived of natural defences by the poor blood supply. The combination of neuropathy, ischaemia and infection leads to chronic indolent sepsis involving the skin, the tissues and the bones. Occlusion of the vascular supply causes ischaemic ulceration of the skin or gangrene, depending on the size of the vessel occluded and the viability of the collateral circulation.

Medial calcification

(Mönckeberg's sclerosis.) This is liable to occur in longstanding diabetes irrespective of age. It is often seen on Xray in the pelvic and limb vessels, and sometimes in the digital vessels, but it does not necessarily impair circulation or function. It is also a feature of diabetic neuropathy.

Microangiopathy

Thickening of the basement membrane of the capillaries, particularly of the glomeruli and retinae but also in many other tissues, has been observed in diabetics by electron microscopy and may be regarded as the hallmark of longstanding diabetes. In general, the degree of thickening is more related to the duration of the diabetes than to any other ascertainable factor. It leads to occlusion of small vessels with ischaemia of tissues involved.

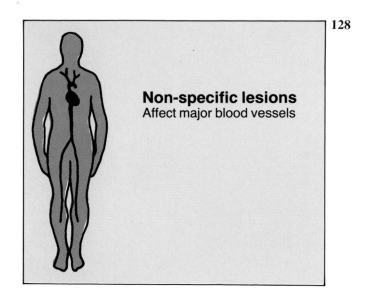

128 Nonspecific disease in major blood vessels.

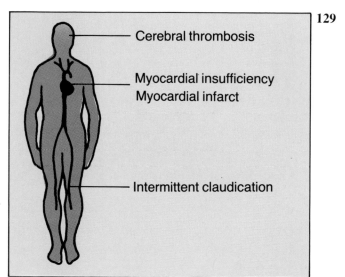

129 Nonspecific vascular disease affecting myocardial, cerebral and lower limb vessels.

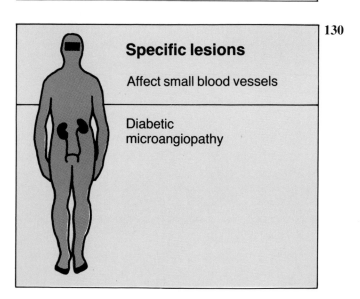

130 Specific diabetic small blood vessel disease (diabetic microangiopathy) clinically evident in retinae, renal glomeruli and lower limb digital capillaries.

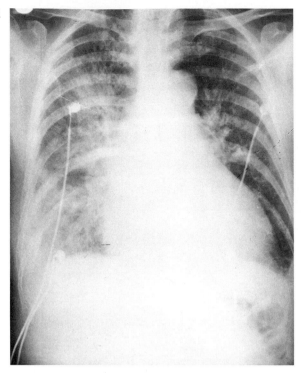

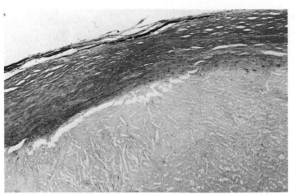

132 Atheromatous plaque in a section of the aorta with a lower pale area of extensive cholesterol deposition. (*MSB × 16*)

131 Cardiomegaly, left heart failure. Pulmonary oedema in a 62-year-old diabetic admitted to an Intensive Care Unit following a recent myocardial infarct. Diabetics (especially females) usually have a worse prognosis and more complications of myocardial infarction than non-diabetics.

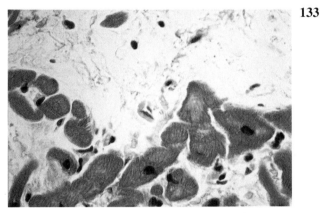

133 A histological section of the myocardium showing an excess of interstitial fibrous tissue. (*H&E × 650*)

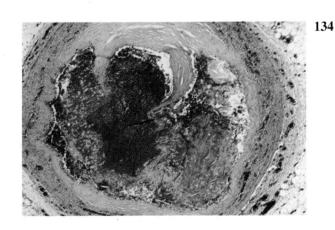

134 Coronary artery occluded by a recent thrombus. (*H&E × 16*)

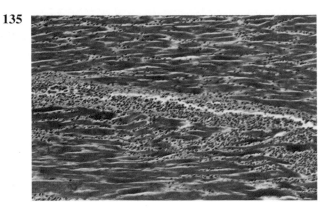

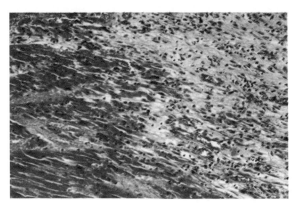

135 Necrotic muscle infiltrated with polymorphs in the myocardium 4 days after infarction. (*H&E × 80*)

136 Early organisation with new vessels, inflammatory cells and fibroblastic connective tissue in the myocardium, 14 days after infarction. (*H&E × 80*)

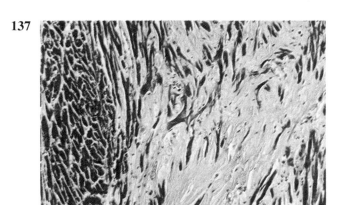

137 Myocardium 3 months after infarction showing extensive pale green connective tissue demonstrated by Masson's trichrome stain. (*× 80*)

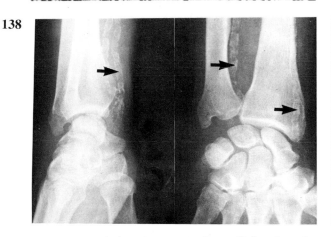

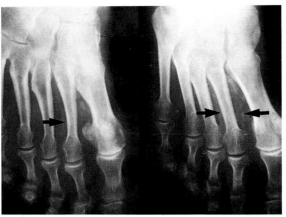

138 Mönckeberg's type of medial sclerosis. Forearm and wrist showing characteristic extensive calcification in the radial and ulnar arteries. Calcification of this severity is especially common in diabetes with renal failure, and it is also a feature of severe neuropathy.

139 Vascular calcification in foot extending into the small plantar arteries (arrowed) in a 48-year-old insulin-dependent diabetic. Vascular calcification is apparent earlier in diabetics and tends to extend into smaller arteries than in non-diabetics. Severe neuropathy may cause medial degeneration and be responsible for medial calcification.

65

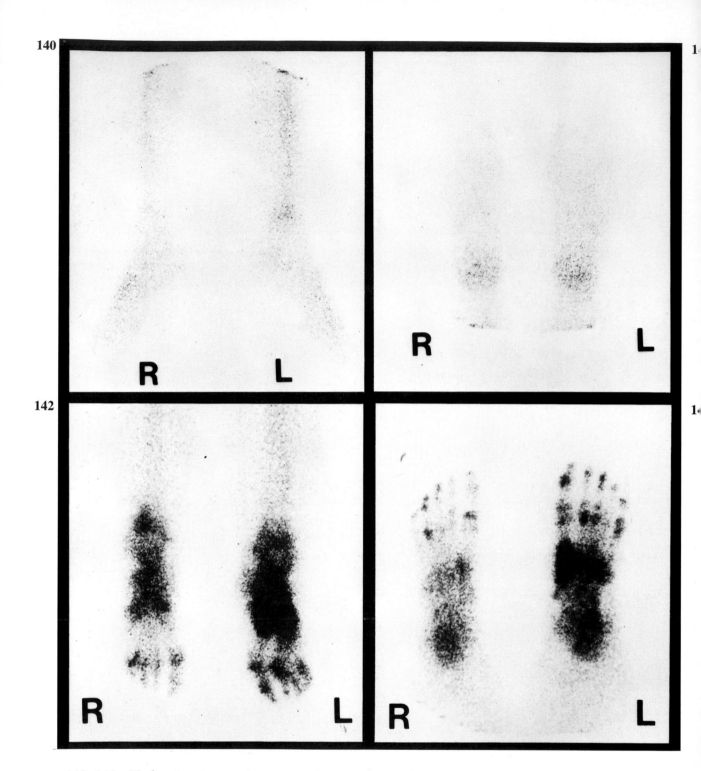

140–143 Technetium isotope bone scans showing the very high uptake in the neuropathic foot (**142** and **143**), compared with the normal foot (**140** and **141**). This high uptake in neuropathy signifies an increase in bone blood flow and occurs before any changes are visible on conventional Xrays.

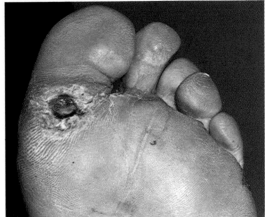

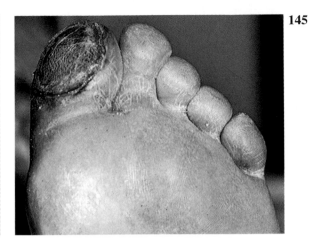

144 Typical neuropathic ulcer at pressure point. Loss of sensation, ischaemia and sepsis all contribute to this lesion in the diabetic. The ulcer is surrounded by callus and is painless. The major arteries are intact.

145 Superficial ischaemic necrosis of a big toe caused by the diabetic patient wearing an ill-fitting shoe. These lesions are superficial, may contain a necrotic base and are painful. The major arteries are impalpable.

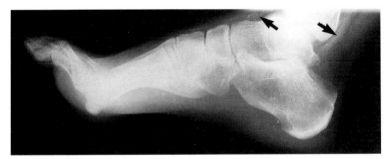

146 Lateral Xray of a neuropathic foot showing clawed toes with prominence of the metatarsal heads; together with medial vascular calcification (arrows) which is a feature of severe peripheral neuropathy in diabetes.

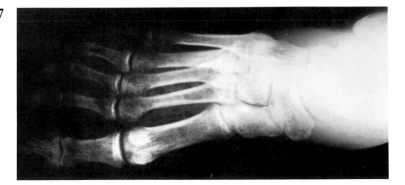

147 Subcutaneous gas in an infected foot is almost pathognomic for diabetes.

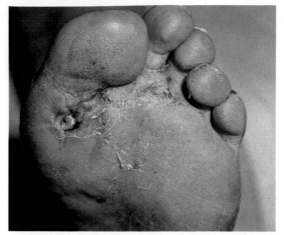

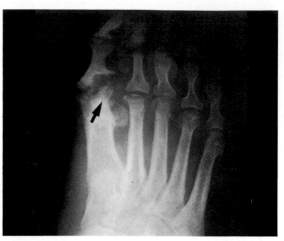

148 Purulent discharging neuropathic ulcer at the base of the big toe, associated with osteomyelitis of the first metatarsal head. Pus must be drained surgically as a matter of urgency, if an abcess develops and does not drain spontaneously.

149 Osteomyelitis. Bony destruction is a serious feature usually requiring excisions by bony amputation.

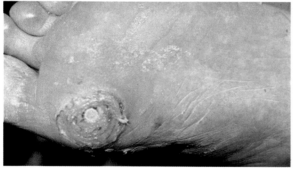

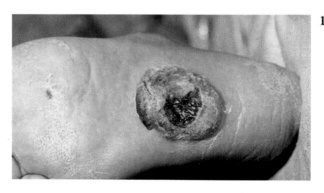

150 Neuropathic ulcer with pronounced hyper-keratosis.

151 Neuropathic ulcer with hyperkeratosis on sole of foot.

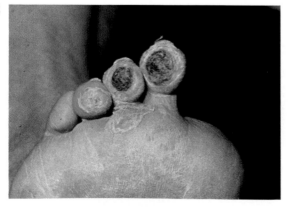

152 Painless destructive damage to neuropathic toes caused by falling asleep when warming feet in front of an electric fire.

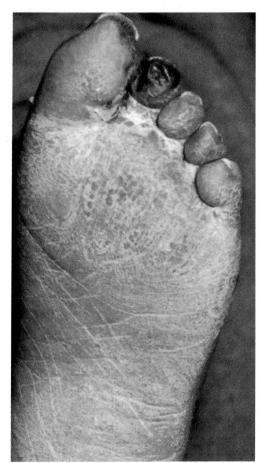

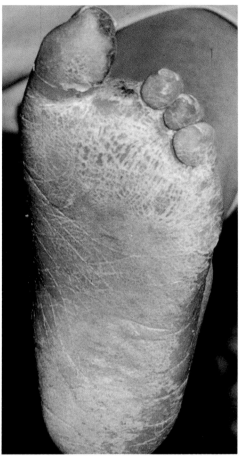

153 Gangrene of second left toe in a neuropathic diabetic.

154 Local amputation of the second left toe in same patient (**153**).

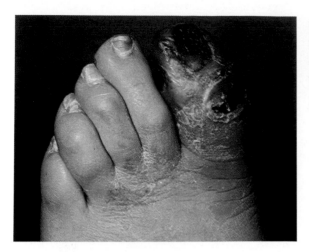

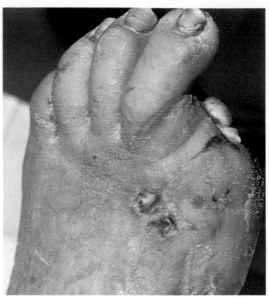

155 Gangrene of a neuropathic left great toe, with a good blood supply to remainder of the foot.

156 Successful amputation in the same patient (**155**). Local operations of this type rarely succeed in the ischaemic foot.

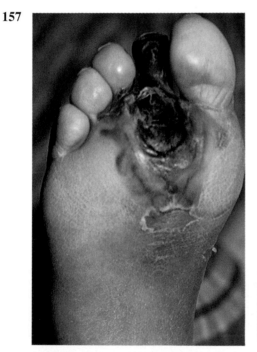

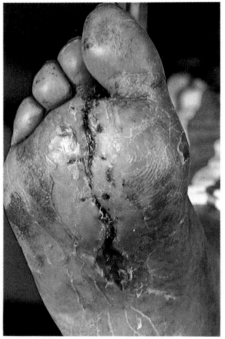

157 Gangrene of the second toe extending to the metatarsal in a neuropathic foot with intact blood supply.

158 Ray excision of the toe and metatarsal in the same patient. Good preservation of function.

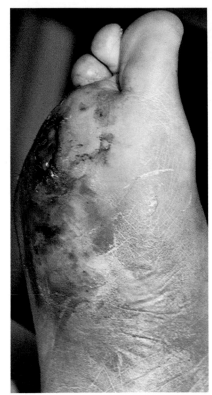

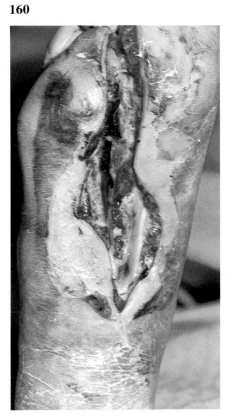

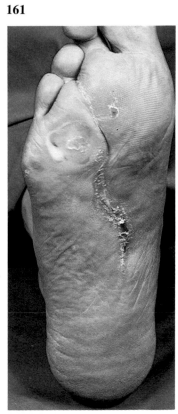

159 Osteomyelitis of the right third metatarsal with deep-tissue cellulitis and pus formation in a neuropathic foot. Diabetes poorly controlled on oral hypoglycaemic agents.

160 Diabetes well controlled by insulin in the same patient (**159**). Ray amputation of middle toe and metatarsal. The circulation was intact.

161 Three months later: same patient (**159**) showing good healing.

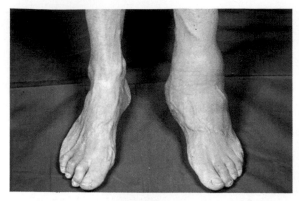 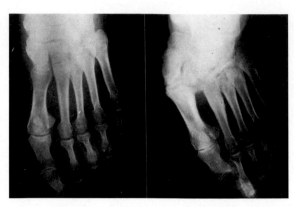

162 Charcot joint of the left foot. Painless distortion and broadening of the left forefoot and ankle. There was little functional disability but the patient had to wear a specially broad shoe on the left foot. On examination, good circulation was noted but sensation and reflexes was absent.

163 Charcot joint of the left foot compared with normal Xray of the same foot taken 5 years earlier. There is now considerable disorganisation of the intertarsal joints.

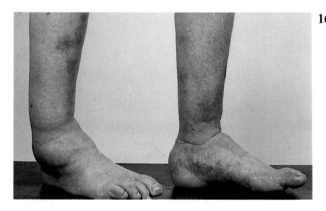

164 Charcot (neuroarthropathic) joints. The feet are grossly deformed from bony destruction and dislocation. The 'rocker' sole is characteristic of this condition.

16

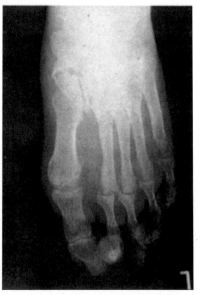

165

165 Radiograph showing the disorganization of the distal joints of the foot.

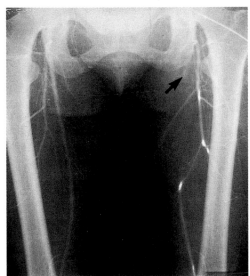

166 Femoral artery occlusion demonstrated on radiograph.

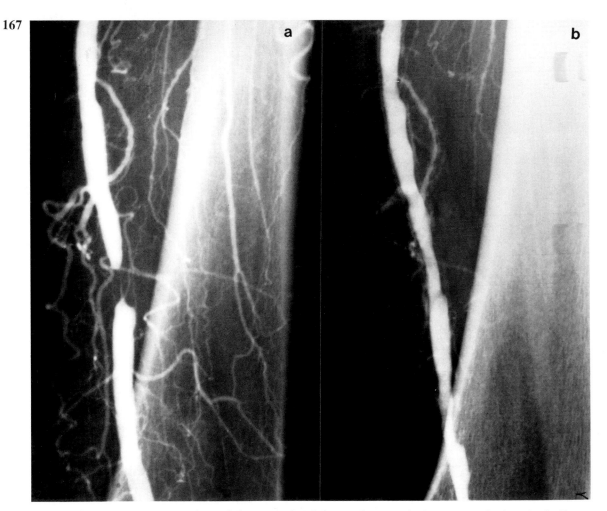

167 **Atheromatous narrowing** of the superficial femoral artery before (a) and after (b) balloon angioplasty.

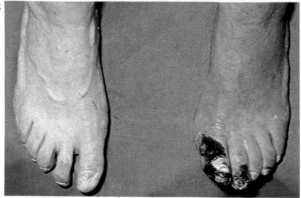

168 **Gangrene** of left first and second toes with ischaemia of leg due to occlusion of deep femoral artery.

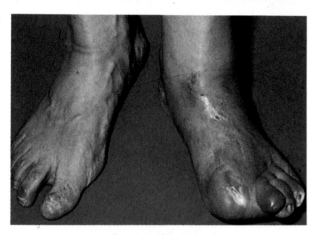

169 **Amputation** and bypass saphenous vein graft carried out in the patient in **168**.

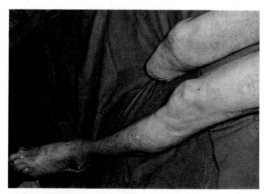

170 **Below-knee amputation** for advanced ischaemic gangrene of the foot: this is the best treatment for extensive gangrene of the foot and permits early fitting of a prosthesis and rehabilitation.

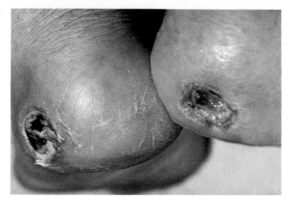

171 **Ulceration of heels** due to pressure of footwear.

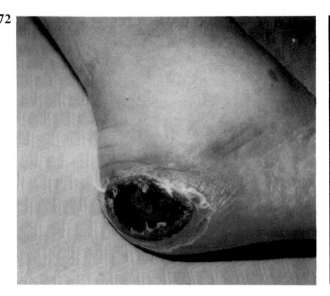

172 Ulceration of heel in a bed-ridden patient whose heels were not protected.

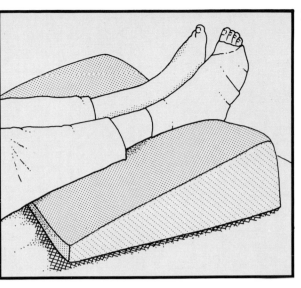

173 Foam wedge used to protect the heels of all diabetics requiring bedrest.

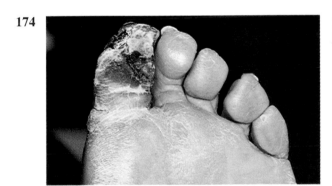

174 Painless ischaemic dry gangrene of the right great toe, unsuspected by mildly diabetic patient.

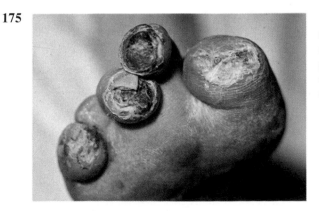

175 Peripheral ischaemia and dry gangrene associated with occlusion of the arcuate vessels of the dorsalis pedis artery. Distal, well localised dry gangrene when limited to digital tips is best treated conservatively; the necrotic areas gradually demarcate and auto-amputate.

8 The skin and connective tissue

Examination of the skin may reveal important information in diabetes. Infection of the skin is common in the untreated patient and insulin may cause changes in the skin and subcutaneous tissues at the site of injections. In longstanding cases of diabetes, metabolic and ischaemic processes may be manifested in the skin.

Infection

Moniliasis

Candida albicans is a yeast which thrives in moist areas of the skin and particularly in uncontrolled diabetes. Thus, when glycosuria is substantial, severe vulvitis occurs in women, and less commonly balanitis in men. The infection often leads to redness, oedema and maceration of the skin and gives rise to intense irritation. Scratching of the area can cause secondary bacterial infection. Inappropriate treatment with steroids or antibiotics can lead to a spread of the monilial infection. Diagnosis should be made by microscopic examination of a scraping for mycelia; the infection usually responds to control of the diabetes and application of appropriate antifungal therapy.

Epidermophytosis

Sometimes known as athlete's foot, this is a common infection occurring between the toes and leading to sogginess and maceration of the skin in the toe clefts. It may also be present in the groins as reddened, moist and irritating areas (tinea cruris).

Bacterial infections of the skin

Boils, carbuncles, impetigo or cellulitis sometimes occur in undiagnosed diabetics. Indeed, routine examination of the urine in such cases often leads to the diagnosis of diabetes. Occasionally lack of hygiene causes infection at the site of insulin injection. Good control of diabetes is of prime importance in these infections; patients taking hypoglycaemic oral agents should be transferred to insulin, if the blood sugars are elevated in the presence of infection.

Vascular

Venous (gravitational) ulceration

This occurs on the skin of the legs usually after minor trauma or it may occur spontaneously. These ulcers may be seen in areas associated with varicose veins; or they may occur on the shins or dorsum of the foot. The ulcers are usually shallow and indolent, and can be very painful.

Diabetic dermopathy

This is the name given to depressed, atrophic and sometimes pigmented rounded areas on the shins of both legs in diabetics, which are probably due to microangiopathy.

Metabolic

Xanthomatosis

Eruptive xanthomata occur in untreated diabetics and the disorder is associated with lipaemia retinalis and hypertriglyceridaemia. The plasma is milky white in colour. The condition rapidly subsides in most cases after the institution of insulin therapy. If it does not, it suggests the presence of an associated hereditary hyperlipidaemia.

Familial hypercholesterolaemia can be associated with diabetes and gives rise to tendon and tuberous xanthomata. Unless triglycerides are also raised, the plasma in these cases is clear. Control of the diabetes in this situation has no effect on the skin lesions. Xanthoma tendinosum occurs as a firm nodular infiltration of the tendon sheaths, often on the extensor tendons of the hands or the tendon Achilles. Tuberous xanthomas develop slowly as fleshy to firm nodules especially on the extensor surfaces of elbows and knees.

Xanthelasma

This is the name given to the raised yellow fatty deposits on the eyelids. The disorder is as common in non-diabetics as in diabetics and does not necessarily denote a systemic disorder, although it is sometimes associated with a lipid disorder.

Necrobiosis lipoidica

This skin disorder may precede the onset of symptomatic diabetes and indeed, its presence may lead to the diagnosis of diabetes. It occurs most commonly on the front of the lower legs but occasionally appears on the upper limbs or the trunk. It starts as raised red papules with a yellowish middle which slowly coalesce and spread. The centre becomes atrophic and is often covered by a silvery scale. Telangiectasis may be seen in the atrophic area. Although the lesions may be indolent and persist for some years, they usually heal spontaneously leaving an area of pigmented scar. The lesions are painless and although unsightly, seldom lead to ulceration. Necrobiosis is commoner in women than in men. The nature of the disorder is not understood. Histologically, there are obliterative lesions in the microvasculature with disintegration of collagen fibres and lipoid deposits.

Skin disorders caused by insulin injections

Abscess formation

Occasionally lack of simple hygiene leads to infection of the site of injections.

Allergy

Because insulin from animal sources is foreign material, local allergic reaction sometimes occurs with the initiation of insulin therapy. Porcine insulin is less antigenic than bovine but with the advent of monocomponent porcine insulin and human insulin, allergic reactions are less common.

Oedema

Retention of fluid sometimes occurs when insulin therapy is started or when the dose is greatly increased. This is normally manifested as oedema of the legs and is probably due to temporary inhibition of sodium excretion.

Lipohypertrophy

Insulin injections sometimes lead to the formation of soft, painless swellings at the site of the injections. These areas of fat hypertrophy are most likely to occur when the same area is used for injections each time. They are less likely to form if varying sites of injection are chosen. They may result in erratic insulin absorption and functions in diabetic control.

Lipoatrophy

This was particularly common in young women and appeared as shallow pits which could become disturbing and unsightly. The cause of this fat atrophy is unknown; it was sometimes be seen in areas other than those in which the injections have been sited, suggesting an indirect effect of insulin. Certainly the pits can be encouraged to fill to the normal contour by using human insulin and by injecting directly into the lipatrophic areas. Lipoatrophy has become extremely rare since the introduction of highly purified insulin.

Miscellaneous skin lesions

Granuloma annulare

This occurs more commonly is diabetics than in non-diabetics. Flattened violaceous nodules appear on the fingers, wrists and feet, often in ring formation.

Stiff hands: Dupuytren's contractures

The flexibility of collagen appears to be reduced in diabetes. Stiffness of the skin and Dupuytren's contractures are frequently seen in the palms of patients with diabetes.

Vitiligo

This is common when diabetes is associated with other autoimmune disorders such as pernicious anaemia, thyroid disease, Addison's disease or alopecia.

Drug rashes

These may rarely occur with the sulphonylureas.

Blistering of the skin

This sometimes develops in patients in diabetic ketoacidosis or prolonged hypoglycaemia, presumably caused by pressure and dehydration. Bullae may also occur without obvious cause in poorly controlled diabetics (*bullosis diabeticorum*).

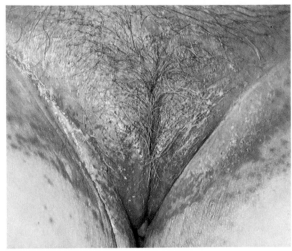

176 **Pruritus vulvae** in newly diagnosed diabetic. Note soggy excoriation of skin due to moniliasis.

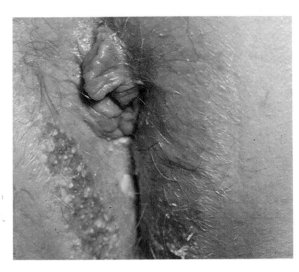

177 **Pruritus ani** associated with epidermophytosis in newly diagnosed diabetic.

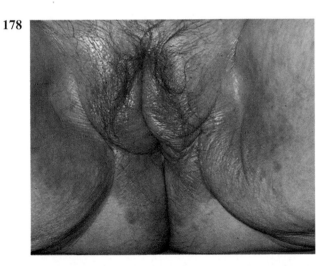

178 **Resolving pruritus vulvae and ani** in recently poorly controlled diabetic.

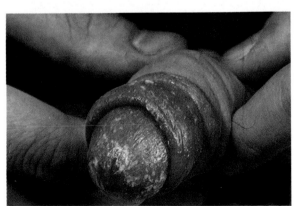

179 **Balanitis** as a presenting feature of diabetes.

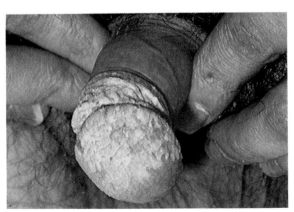

180 **Balanitis** due to candidiasis in poorly controlled diabetes.

181 Intertrigenous **candidiasis** below both breasts.

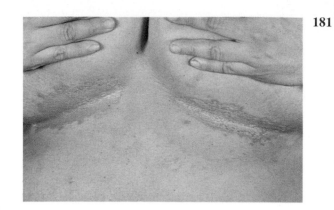

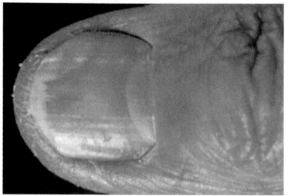

182 **Nail changes with lateral onycholysis,** thining of nail plate and growth arrest lines in a 72-year-old diabetic with long-standing requirement for insulin.

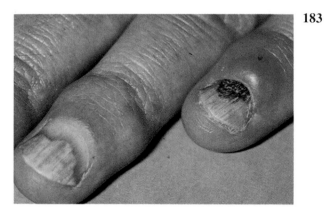

183 **Moniliasis** of fingernails.

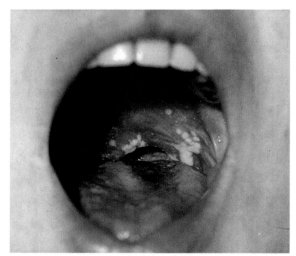

184 **Throat infection** in a diabetic, treated with antibiotics and causing oral candidiasis.

185 Herpes zoster involving ophthalmic division of left fifth cranial nerve. Herpes zoster is particularly common in diabetics.

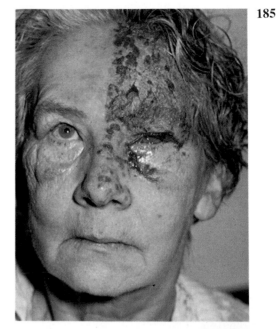

186 Pyogenic infections such as boils, furuncles and staphylococcal carbuncles can occur in poorly controlled diabetes.

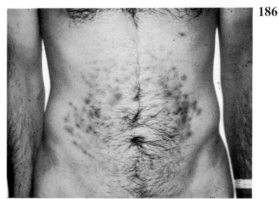

187 Carbuncle on neck can be the presenting feature in maturity-onset diabetics. Any patient with skin infection should be suspected of diabetes.

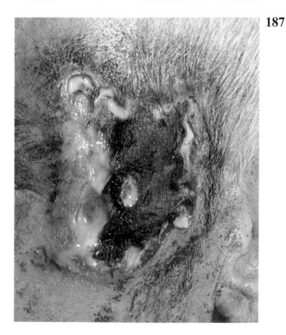

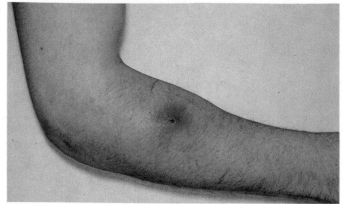

188 Furuncle on forearm in poorly controlled diabetic.

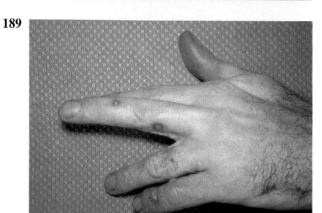

189 Multiple furuncles on the hand of a diabetic.

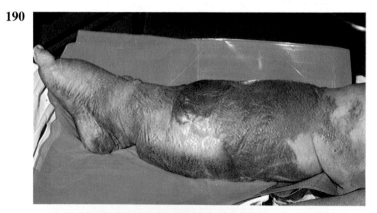

190 Cellulitis of leg in an elderly diabetic, associated with deep-vein thrombosis.

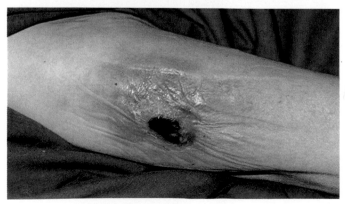

191 Sepsis at site of insulin injection following lack of cleanliness in injection technique and poorly controlled diabetes. Such lesions are relatively unusual.

192 Septic pulp in young diabetic girl who had been using the finger to test her own blood sugars. This complication is surprisingly rare.

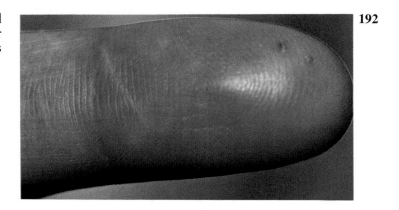

192

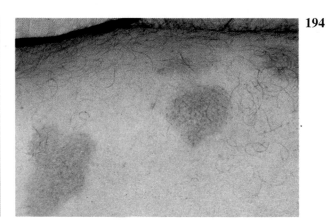

193

193 Local allergy to insulin injections. Hot irritating erythematous areas.

194

194 Insulin allergy in the thigh.

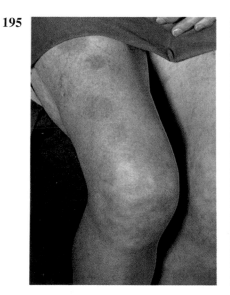

195

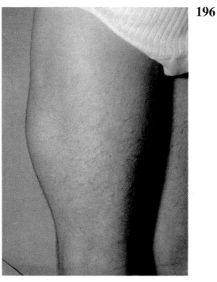

196

195 Extensive local allergy to beef insulin.

196 Lipohypertrophy at site of insulin injection in a male diabetic. The cause is unknown.

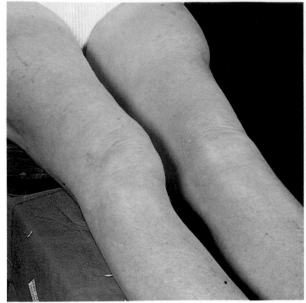

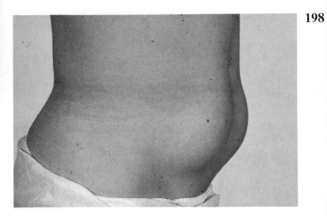

197 Lipohypertrophy at site of insulin injection in the thighs of female patient.

198 Lipohypertrophy in lower abdomen in young female diabetic.

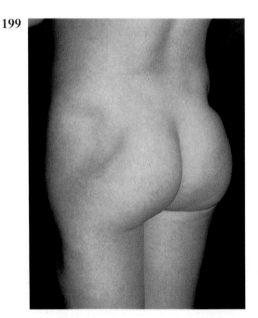

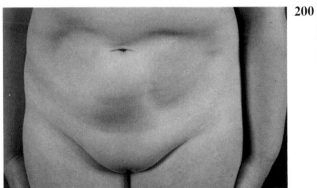

199 Lipoatrophy over buttocks and thighs at site of insulin injections in a young female.

200 Lipoatrophy at abdominal injection sites in an adolescent diabetic.

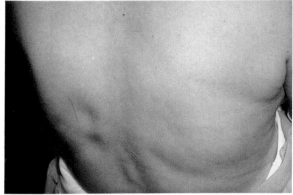

201 Lipoatrophy of the back in a patient given injections into the back by her husband.

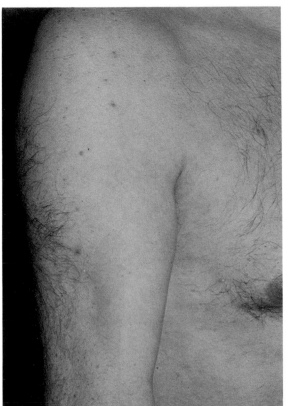

202 Lipoatrophy in the upper arm following insulin injections.

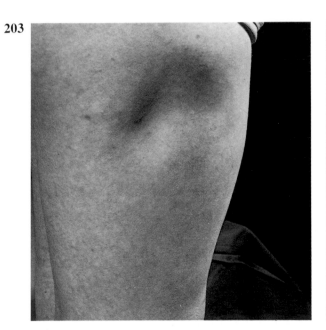

203 Lipoatrophy in the thigh of young woman at site of insulin injections.

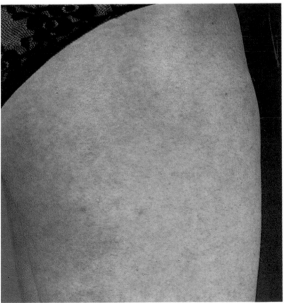

204 Atrophic area restored to normal in same patient (**203**) after 6 weeks by changing to highly purified insulin and injecting into atrophic site.

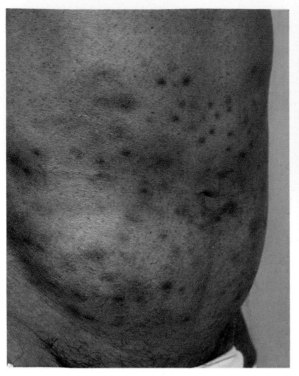

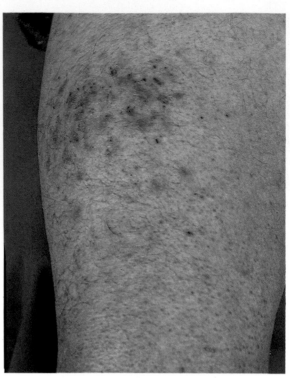

205 Superficial lesions in the abdomen resulting from *intradermal* injection of insulin. Intradermal injections are painful and injections should be subcutaneous.

206 Superficial lesions similar to 205 in the thigh, stressing the importance of injecting insulin subcutaneously and not intradermally.

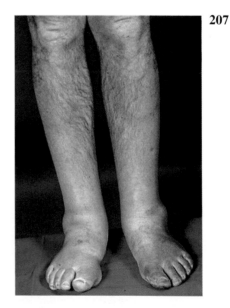

207 Lower limb oedema following increased insulin dose in previously poorly controlled diabetic. Insulin can lead to temporary inhibition of salt excretion with fluid retention, but this usually subsides spontaneously.

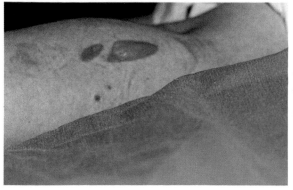

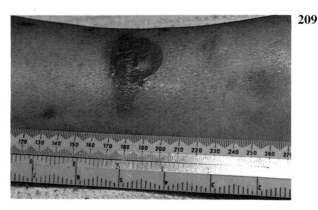

208 **Bullous lesions** on back of calf in a young woman recovering from a diabetic coma, probably due to a combination of pressure and dehydration.

209 **Bullous lesion** similar to **208** in a male patient recovering from a diabetic coma.

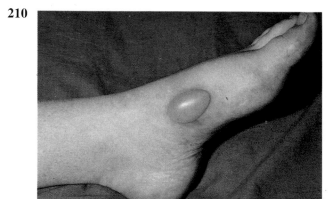

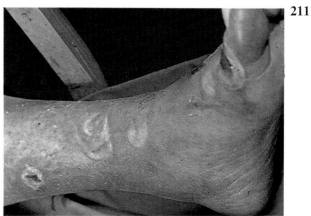

210 **Bulla on the foot** of a young diabetic girl recovering from hypoglycaemic coma.

211 **Bullosis diabeticorum.** Spontaneously occurring bullae in a poorly controlled diabetic.

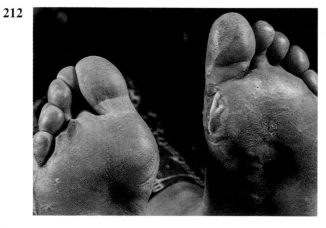

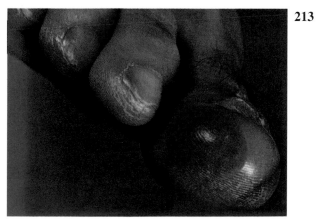

212 and **213** **Bullosis diabeticorum** involving the toes.

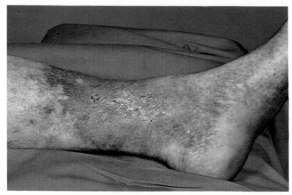

214 **Varicose eczema** in a diabetic.

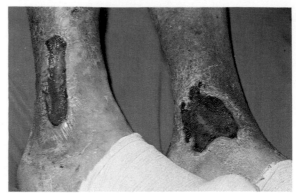

215 **Martorell's ulceration.** Ischaemic ulcers in a diabetic with hypertension. These ulcers are caused by avascular skin necrosis and do not appear in pressure areas. They may develop very rapidly.

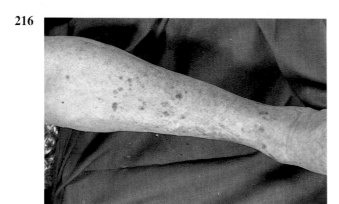

216 **Diabetic dermopathy:** scattered pigmented atrophic lesions on the shins.

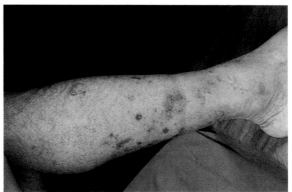

217 **Scattered and confluent lesions** similar to 216.

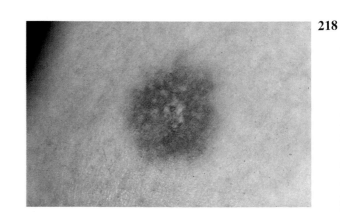

218 **Necrobiosis lipoidica diabeticorum:** early lesion showing yellow papules.

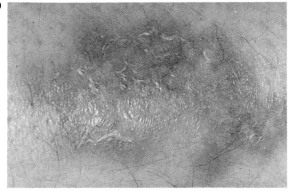

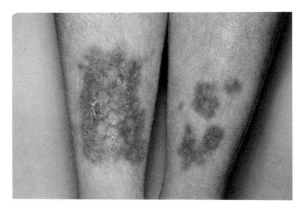

219 **Necrobiosis lipoidica diabeticorum** show-ing silvery surface scales.

220 **Necrobiosis lipoidica diabeticorum** on shins with some central ulceration.

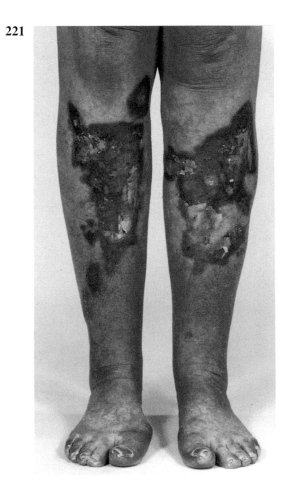

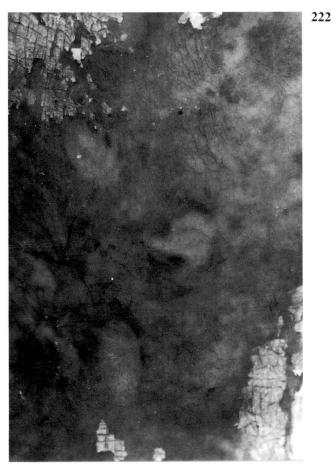

221 and 222 **Necrobiosis lipoidica diabeticorum.** These rare but disfiguring lesions develop on the shins of diabetic patients, and only occur occasionally elsewhere. They show an atrophic telangiectatic centre, which can ulcerate, surrounded by a slight raised pinkish margin.

223

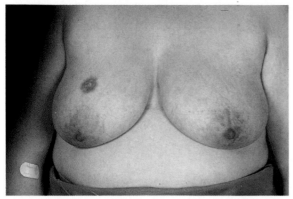

223 Necrobiosis lipoidica diabeticorum: an unusual site over the breast in an unsuspected diabetic. The lesion gave rise to the diagnosis.

224

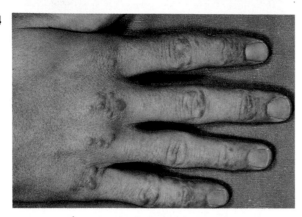

224 Granuloma annulare on the hand. This skin disorder is often associated with diabetes.

225

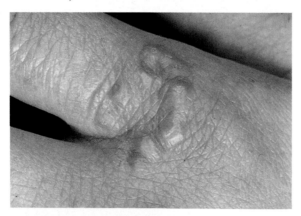

225 Granuloma annulare in close-up on a finger showing ring formation.

226

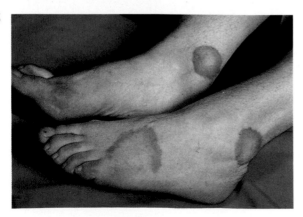

226 Granuloma annulare in a diabetic woman, occurring on the feet, another common site.

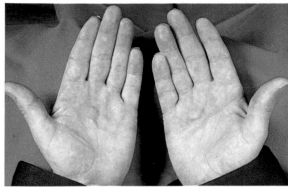

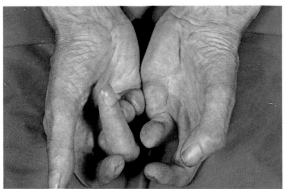

227 Early Dupuytren's contracture in a diabetic.

228 Dupuytren's contracture: a severe example of a common disorder in diabetics.

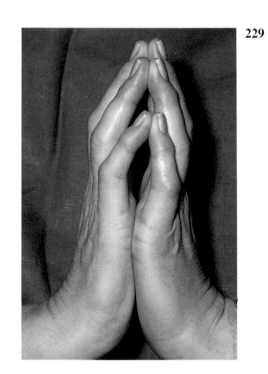

229

229 Stiff hands in a diabetic. Hands in the praying position, unable to flatten palms together. This condition is known as cheiroarthropathy: it may be due to collagen degeneration, and is symptomless.

230

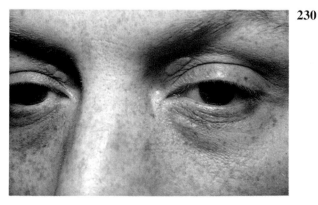

230 Xanthelasma in a diabetic. This local lesion was not associated with any known constitutional lipid abnormality, although it can be associated with hypercholesterolaemia.

231

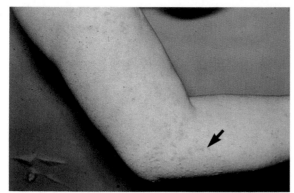

231 **Eruptive xanthomata** associated with uncontrolled diabetes.

232

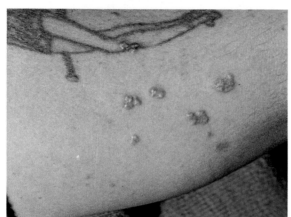

232 **Eruptive xanthomata** showing characteristic discrete firm bright yellow papules surrounded by a red rim. These are associated with very severe hyperlipidaemia leading to a milky plasma and lipaemia retinalis which very rarely occurs in uncontrolled diabetes.

233

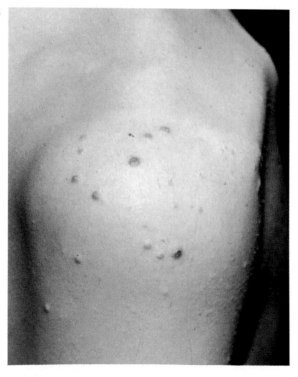

233 **Eruptive xanthomata** in a newly diagnosed diabetic girl, disappearing within a few weeks of insulin therapy.

234

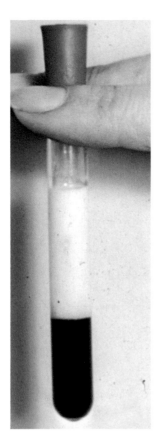

234 **Eruptive xanthomata.** Milky serum from 233 before treatment and returning to normal after insulin.

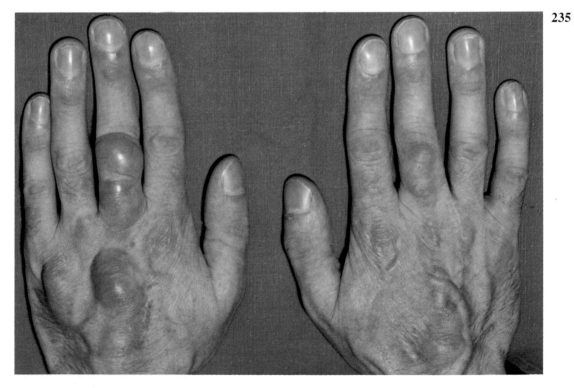

235

235 **Xanthomata tendinosum,** firm nodules attached to extensor tendons and associated with familial hypercholesterolaemia.

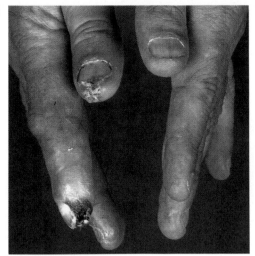

236

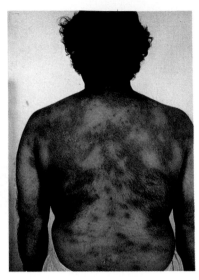

237

236 Gangrene of fingertip. Digital artery thrombosis sometimes occurs in diabetes in renal failure, especially if there is fistula or shunt.

237 Pseudoxanthoma nigricans. This condition is seen particularly in obese diabetics. The dusky, pigmented, hyperkeratotic lesions affect the axillae, groins and skin folds round the neck resembling true acanthosis nigricans. This condition is associated with insulin resistance and polycystic ovaries.

238

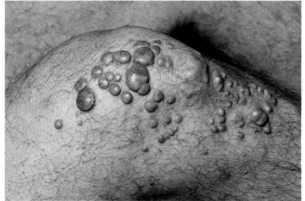

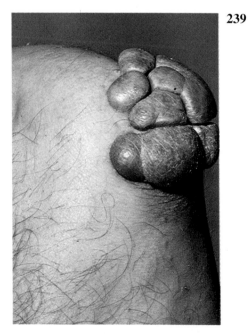

239

238 Tuberous xanthomata associated with hypercholesterolaemia. These growths are located in the skin but are not attached to underlying tissues and unaffected by insulin therapy.

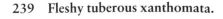

239 Fleshy tuberous xanthomata.

240 Necrotizing external otitis. Necrotizing external otitis (malignant external otitis) is a rare infection of the temporal bone due to *Pseudomonas aeruginosa*. It is seen typically in elderly diabetics and is characterised by granulation tissue and necrosis in the external auditory canal.

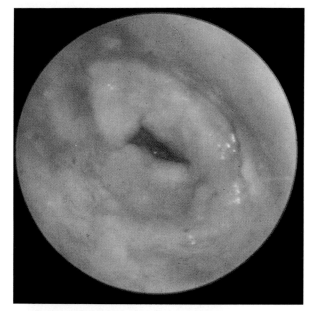

241 'Malignant' otitis externa is a rare and serious form of otitis externa to which elderly diabetics are particularly susceptible. Granulation tissue is found in the meatus infected with pseudomonas and anaerobic organisms. This granulation tissue tends to erode deeply to involve the middle and inner ear, the bone of the skull base, with extension to the brain and also the great vessels of the neck. Intense antibiotic therapy often associated with surgical drainage of the affected areas is necessary. It is not a 'malignant' condition in the histological sense for the biopsies of granulation tissue show inflammatory changes only; 'necrotizing' otitis externa may be more accurate, but 'malignant' indicates the serious clinical nature.

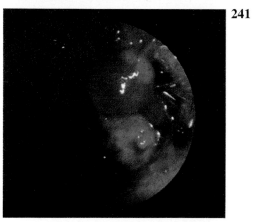

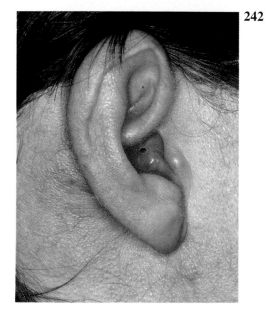

242 'Deep' otitis externa. An uncommon form of otitis externa involves predominantly the skin of the deep bony meatus and the surface of the tympanic membrane. The drum epithelium may become replaced with sessile granulations infected with *Pseudomonas pyocyanea*. In protracted cases of this type of otitis externa the skin of the deep meatus and drum becomes thickened and 'funnelled' with meatal atresia. The resulting conductive hearing loss is extremely difficult to treat surgically once this condition is quiescent.

9 The nervous system

Peripheral polyneuropathy

Pathology

Patchy loss of myelin segments (segmental demyelination) is the fundamental histological lesion in diabetic neuropathy. The myelin sheath arises as an outgrowth of the Schwann cell, but it is uncertain whether the demyelination is caused by a defect in the Schwann cell or by primary disease in the axon. In the early stages of neuropathy the axons remain intact, allowing remyelination and recovery. In more advanced cases, the axons fragment and remyelination does not occur.

Chronic hyperglycaemia can be shown to alter metabolism in peripheral nerves with accumulation of sorbitol resulting from a diversion of glucose in the sorbitol-fructose pathway. Uncertainty remains regarding the precise aetiology of diabetic neuropathy because in addition to metabolic factors, several vascular anomalies have also been identified. Thrombotic lesions have been demonstrated in the small intraneural and perineural blood vessels and platelet behaviour is abnormal.

Clinical features

Symptoms of neuropathy may occur in the untreated diabetic and are probably caused by the elevated blood sugar. Paraesthesia in the extremities, pain or numbness in the feet and the calves may be presenting symptoms in the newly diagnosed diabetic and usually disappear with the initiation of treatment and restoration to normoglycaemia.

Much more permanent are the features of neuropathy associated with longstanding diabetes. Loss of sensation is common, particularly in the feet but also in the hands, and can be associated with troublesome paraesthesia or deep-seated pain, particularly at night, in the legs. There may be wasting of the small muscles of the hands and feet. The reflexes in the legs are reduced or absent. There is a loss of sensation to cotton wool and pin prick, and vibration sense is impaired. Deep pain sensation is lost. Changes secondary to this neuropathy are normally evident. The hair is lost over the lower two-thirds of the leg, small atrophic pits occur in the skin of the legs (dermopathy) and indolent neuropathic painless ulcers frequently are present on the soles of the feet.

In severe cases, the loss of proprioceptive pathways leads to sensory ataxia with unsteadiness of gait, sometimes referred to as pseudo-tabes and often made worse by deterioration of vision.

Diabetic amyotrophy (femoral neuropathy, proximal motor neuropathy)

This form of neuropathy affects mainly the motor fibres. It occurs most commonly in older males and is often associated with intolerable persistent pain. The proximal muscles of the legs are most involved, sometimes the shoulder muscles as well. Weakness and wasting may be so profound that the patient is unable to walk. These features may be superimposed on a diabetic of longstanding already with neuropathy: or they may arise in a case of recent onset, particularly if the diabetes is poorly controlled.

The physical findings are variable. The reflexes are usually lost, there is a variable sensory loss. Wasting of the muscles, especially the quadriceps, may be associated with fasciculation and the plantar responses are sometimes extensor.

Although the disorder may persist for many weeks or even months, most patients make a slow recovery with lessening pain and increasing strength in the limbs. Clearly the diabetes should be kept as well controlled as possible, although it is by no means certain that good control is responsible for improvement.

Mononeuropathy

Individual nerves are commonly involved in diabetes. Of the cranial nerves, the sixth nerve is most frequently affected, sometimes the third nerve and sometimes both. The presenting features are diplopia and squint.

Lesions of the peripheral nerves can give rise to weakness, wasting, pain and sensory loss appropriate to the nerve involved. The ulnar nerve is often affected with wasting of the small muscles of the hand. Other nerves commonly involved include the median, femoral and sciatic, sometimes with manifestations mainly sensory, sometimes motor. The thoracic nerves can also be affected in diabetes (truncal mononeuropathy), and although sensory symptoms usually predominate, unilateral bulging of the abdominal wall may occur.

Functional recovery is the rule with mononeuropathy but it may be slow and incomplete.

Charcot's joints in diabetes are typified by the site of involvement, this being nearly always the intertarsal joints and less commonly the tarsometatarsal joints, the metatarsophalangeal joints and the ankle joints. Involvement in these areas is pathognomonic of diabetes and differentiates it from the Charcot joints occurring in tabes (affecting the knees) and syringomyelia (shoulders and elbows). Xray shows disintegration of the joints, with erosion of the bones and loss of joint space. Clinically, the foot becomes shorter and wider with loss of the arch and a tendency to eversion. Although this deformity necessitates the wearing of surgical boots and makes walking ungainly, the condition is painless and mobility is not materially affected.

Autonomic neuropathy

Widespread involvement of the autonomic system may occur in longstanding diabetes, usually associated with peripheral neuropathy.

Cardiovascular system

Postural hypotension can often be detected in diabetes, and occasionally is severe enough to cause unpleasant symptoms of faintness and dizziness on standing, often assumed by the patient to be a hypoglycaemic reaction. For reasons not clearly understood, the blood pressure may fall shortly after injections of insulin.

Autonomic denervation of the heart may be detected by various simple tests. There is failure of response to the Valsalva manoeuvre; a forced expiration with nose and mouth closed fails to cause any change in the heart rate or blood pressure. A sustained and measured hand grip fails to lead to a normal rise in blood pressure. The normal heart shows a variation of interval between heart beats; this variation is lost in diabetics with cardiac denervation (see **Table 6**). More importantly, in practice autonomic denervation may mean the heart cannot respond to stress. Diabetics with ischaemic heart disease seem less likely to get angina than non-diabetics similarly affected, and this may explain the occasional sudden death occurring in diabetics.

Table 6. Denervated diabetic heart

Persistent tachycardia

Fixed heart rate

Inability to increase cardiac output

Hypotension induced by standing or exercise

Loss of angina pain, painless coronary thrombosis

Gastrointestinal tract

Oesophageal atony and delayed gastric emptying are characteristic of the barium meal in longstanding diabetes; these features may be responsible for bouts of vomiting, particularly unwelcome in diabetics because vomiting may provoke keto-acidosis. Indeed, gastroparesis is often associated with ketoacidosis and most cases of diabetic coma are ushered in by vomiting and stomach dilatation.

Diabetic enteropathy is characterised by intermittent diarrhoea, usually occurring at night as well as during the daytime. During the acute stages as many as 20 loose stools may be passed during the day and, especially in the elderly diabetic, faecal incontinence may occur at night. The diarrhoea may persist for several weeks but despite the distressing nature of the bowel disorder, the patient may not look ill or show constitutional disorders. Not all cases of diarrhoea in diabetics are due to autonomic neuropathy. Chronic pancreatitis and the malabsorption syndrome are not uncommon causes of diarrhoea in diabetes.

Skin

Disturbances of the sweating pattern may be associated with diabetic neuropathy, often with areas of anhidrosis. Less commonly, profuse perspiration of the head and neck occurs after eating cheese or curry, the so-called gustatory sweating.

Bladder dysfunction

Studies of bladder dysfunction in diabetics of long duration show that poor emptying of the bladder after micturition is relatively common and may lead to urinary retention. Stasis of urine disposes to infection and can be a cause of pyelonephritis.

The patient may notice a poor stream and infrequent micturition with frequency, urgency and dribbling when infection supervenes. An asymptomatic enlargement of the bladder may be found on manual examination of the abdomen. This may well suggest an enlarged prostate and in elderly patients the two conditions may co-exist.

Impotence

This condition is common after 20 years of diabetes, probably as a result of involvement of the parasympathetic fibres responsible for maintaining an erection. In most cases libido is unaffected and spermatogenesis is normal, although retrograde ejaculation may occur.

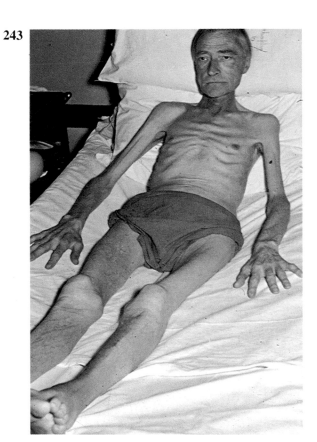

243 Diabetic amyotrophy. The patient complained of pain and weakness in the thighs. He was unable to walk and the diabetes was poorly controlled.

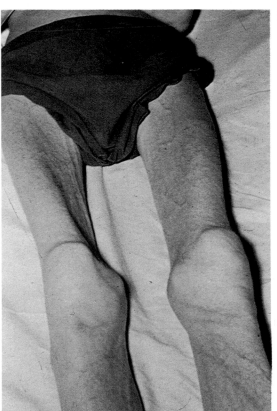

244 Diabetic amyotrophy. Wasted quadriceps muscles (from **243**). Knee jerks were absent. Slow recovery is the rule if the diabetes is properly controlled.

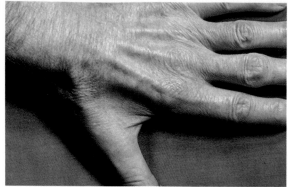

245 Ulnar mononeuropathy. Wasting of the small muscles of the hand in a diabetic, usual due to ulnar nerve compression at the elbow. This rarely causes symptoms.

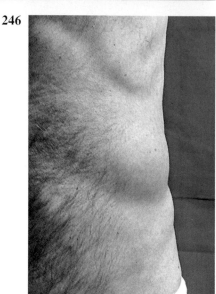

246 Truncal mononeuropathy involving eighth thoracic nerve. Bulging of the lateral abdominal wall in a diabetic.

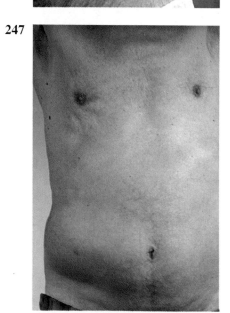

247 Truncal mononeuropathy. Eleventh thoracic nerve palsy with bulging lower abdominal wall. Recovery is the rule.

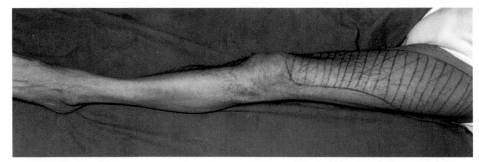

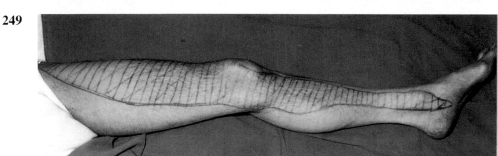

248 and 249 **Diabetic radiculopathy** area of exquisite contact sensitivity can easily and reproducibly traced with a finger – shown in red.

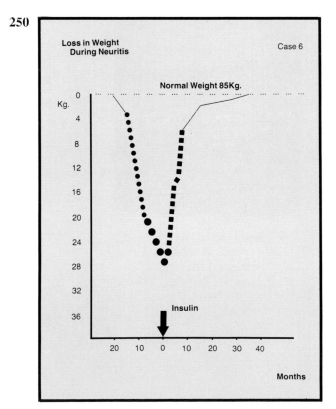

250 **The loss of weight in painful diabetic neuropathy** can be profound, and has led to the description 'diabetic neuropathic cachexia'. Weight loss increases as pain increases (●●●) and returns as pain diminishes (■■■).

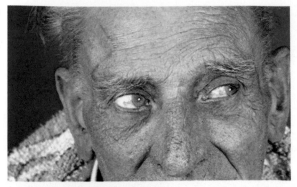

251 Diplopia. Partial third-nerve palsy in the left eye in a diabetic man. Presenting symptom was diplopia. No double vision on looking to the left.

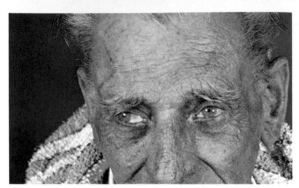

252 Diplopia on looking to the right because the left eye cannot move inward. Good recovery was achieved after 2 months.

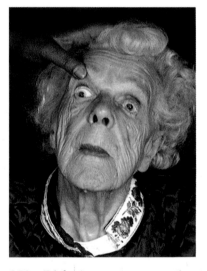

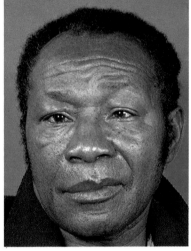

253 Diabetic mononeuropathy. Right third nerve paralysis in an elderly diabetic woman. The right eye is deviated down and outwards. Good recovery can be expected in about 3 months.

254 Right sixth nerve palsy. Double vision on looking to the right because the right eye cannot turn outward. Good recovery of both lesions was achieved after 2 months.

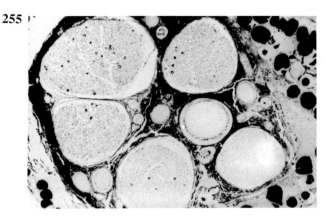

255 Extensive demyelination of the majority of the axons in a cross-section of the sural nerve in a longstanding diabetic. (*Electron micrograph × 500*)

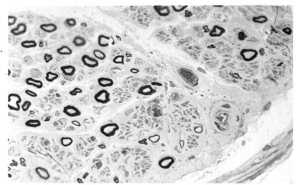

256 Chronic diabetic sensory polyneuropathy. Sural nerve biopsy shows nerve fibre loss. Transverse section of the nerve showing severe loss of myelinated nerve fibres. (*Thionin-acridine orange × 80*)

257

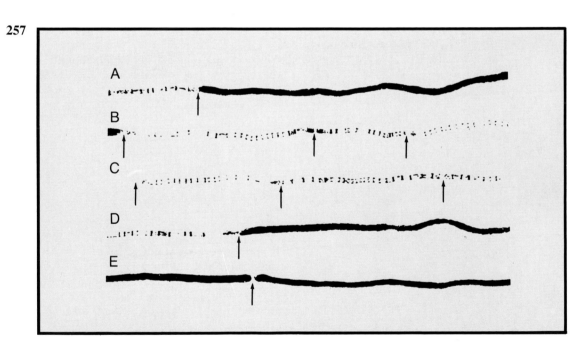

257 Diabetic neuropathy. Segmental demyelination. Isolated nerve fibre from the common peroneal nerve in a patient with diabetic neuropathy. The right hand end of A is continuous with the left hand end of B and similarly from B to E. The nodes of Ranvier are indicated by arrows. The fibre shows preserved segments of thick myelin with intervening remyelinated segments with thin myelin. The darker transverse bands are Schmidt-Lanterman incisures. (*Osmium tetroxide × 500*)

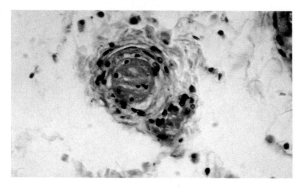

258 Diabetic neuropathy. Sural nerve biopsy showing a thrombosed vessel. The frequent finding of vascular lesions associated with peripheral nerve damage suggests that small blood vessel disease of diabetes may be of aetiological significance. (× 300)

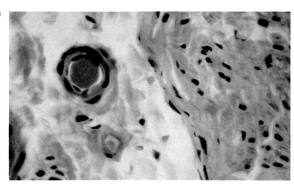

259 Diabetic neuropathy. Sural nerve biopsy showing a ball of organised thrombus in a small blood vessel alongside peripheral nerve tissue. (× 300)

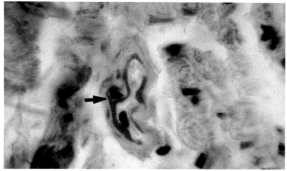

260 Diabetic neuropathy. Sural nerve biopsy showing a small blood vessel lined with fibrin, which can be seen tracking into the vessel wall (arrowed). Thus, fibrin deposition may be of pathogenic significance in diabetic neuropathy. (× 300)

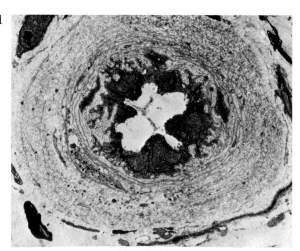

261 Endoneurial capillary from a sural nerve biopsy from a patient having diabetic neuropathy. The endoneurial cells are surrounded by multiple layers of reduplicated basement membrane and associated fibrils. (*Electron micrograph × 1200*)

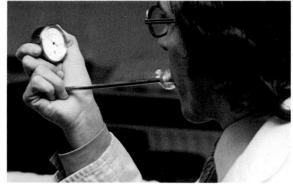 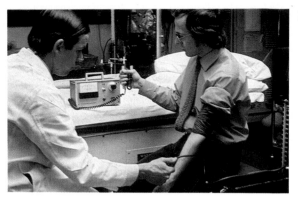

262 **Valsalva manoeuvre** in the diagnosis of diabetic autonomic neuropathy. Subject blows into mouthpiece and maintains pressure of 40mm on manometer for 15 seconds. Heart rate recorded on continuous electrocardiogram. Normal subjects show sinus bradycardia but the rate remains unchanged in diabetic cardiac denervation.

263 **Test for autonomic neuropathy.** Sustained hand grip for up to 5 minutes. In autonomic neuropathy the diastolic blood pressure fails to rise to the normal extent.

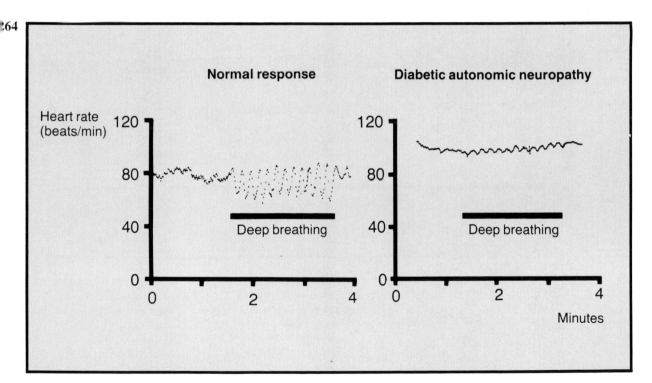

264 **Absence of beat-to-beat heart rate** variation on deep breathing in diabetic autonomic neuropathy, compared to normal. This is due to cardiac vagal denervation. The average heart rate difference (maximum minus minimum at the end of each breath) over six breaths in one minute is recorded. In those under 60 years of age, the normal value is greater than 15, abnormal less than 10.

Table 7. Normal values for autonomic function tests*

	Normal	Abnormal
Heart rate variation (deep breathing)	>15	<10
Heart rate on standing (at 15 seconds)	>15	<12
Heart rate on standing 30:15 ratio	>1.04	<1.00
Valsalva ratio	>1.21	<1.20
Postural systolic pressure fall at 2 minutes	<10mmHg	>30mmHg

*These tests decline with age. The figures given here apply generally in those less than 60 years of age.

265

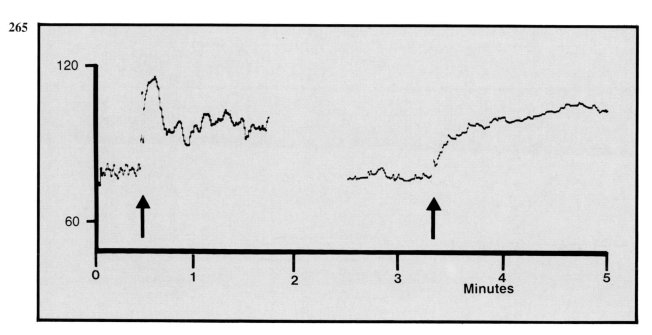

265 **Autonomic neuropathy.** Heart rate changes on standing: normally the effect of standing from the lying position is to cause an overshoot of heart rate, and effect which is lost in autonomic neuropathy, together with a progressive reduction in heart-rate acceleration at 15 seconds.

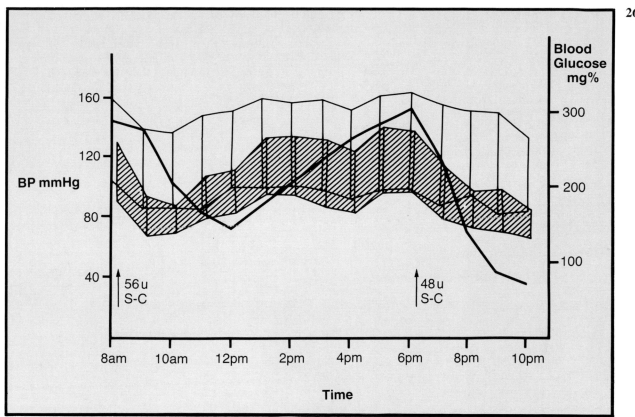

266 Postural hypotension fluctuates through the day and night. In this case the hypotension worsened after insulin injection. Loss of consciousness from this cause can occasionally be confused with hypoglycaemia.

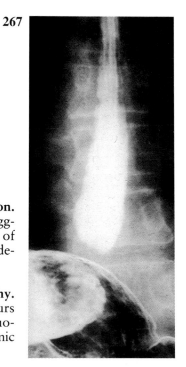

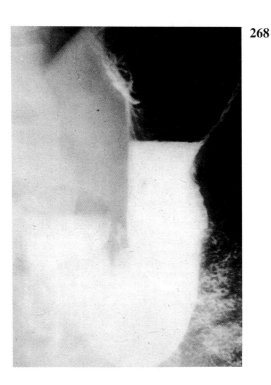

267 Autonomic denervation. Barium swallow showing sluggish contractions and dilatation of oesophagus due to autonomic denervation.

268 Autonomic neuropathy. Barium in the stomach 3 hours after ingestion. Gastric and duodenal atony in diabetic autonomic neuropathy.

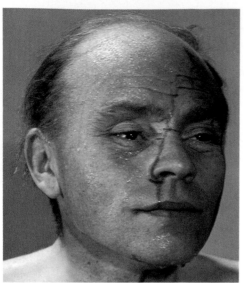

269 Autonomic neuropathy. Gustatory sweating: marked facial sweating in a diabetic, following a meal especially stimulated by spices and cheese. Purple discoloration caused by iodide applied to the face to outline the distribution of the response.

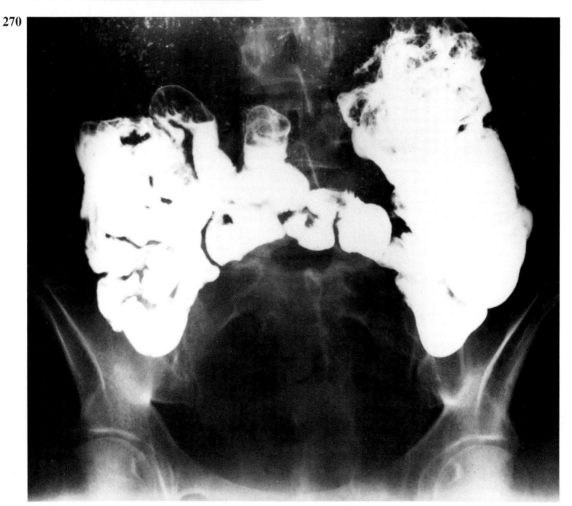

270 Bladder distension resulting from a neurogenic bladder is seen here during a barium follow-through examination.

10 The eye

Diabetic retinopathy is the commonest medical cause of blindness in Britain (**Table 8**). Successful treatment, especially using photocoagulation, can now delay or prevent blindness in many cases so that careful ophthalmoscopic examination of the diabetic patient, at regular intervals, has become increasingly important. Ophthalmoscopy is also valuable because the retina provides an easily accessible indication of the state of small blood-vessel disease elsewhere. The finding of retinopathy is a clinical indication to the patient also having microangiopathy in renal vessels (Chapter 11) and elsewhere.

Although the aetiology and pathogenesis of diabetic retinopathy are not yet clearly understood, several defects probably underlie its development: *capillary closure; alteration in the blood-retinal barrier; abnormal retinal metabolism; and neovascularisation in response to hypoxia.*

Table 8. Diabetic eye disease in Britain

8000 registered blind diabetics

2% diabetics are blind

Diabetes is the commonest cause of blindness in 30-65 age group (15.7%)

80% diabetics have retinopathy after 20 years of diabetes

Capillary closure is the earliest lesion which has been demonstrated both experimentally and by fluorescein angiography. Areas of closure of non-perfusion are usually patchy and occur at the arteriolar end of capillaries where microaneurysms develop simultaneously.

Capillary damage with loss of pericytes may cause a breach in the blood-retinal barrier allowing leakage of lipid and other macromolecules leading to exudate formation.

The retina has a high oxygen demand, and when capillary flow is impaired, altered metabolism in the retinal tissue with local production of lactic acid or other metabolites may be associated with retinal swelling and occlusion of venous flow. Venous irregularity and dilation are both characteristic of diabetic retinopathy.

Retinal hypoxia is the main stimulus to retinal new vessel formation, whether arising from capillary closure or altered venous flow. Abnormal new vessels, especially when growing forwards into the vitreous, are liable to extensive haemorrhage which, together with the fibrous repair reaction stimulated thereafter in the vitreous, then becomes the major threat to vision.

Although poor diabetic control and abnormal growth hormone secretion have both been implicated in the above processes, their precise effects remain speculative. From the clinical standpoint, however, *duration of diabetes* is the single factor which correlates best with retinopathy. Thus, the longer the duration of diabetes, especially in the insulin-dependent type of more than 15 years duration, the greater the likelihood of retinopathy being present and the need for regular expert surveillance.

Although most attention focuses upon the retina, lesions of any of the ocular tissues can be found in diabetes mellitus. Moreover, pathology in these other parts of the eye may often lead the patient to seek medical advice, thus bringing the diagnosis of diabetes to light. Examination of the following systems can be a valuable prelude to a detailed view of the fundus: lids and conjunctivae; eye muscles; anterior uvea; lens opacities; and intra-ocular tension and glaucoma.

Lids and conjunctivae

Often the previously undiagnosed diabetic patient presents with styes or blepharo-conjunctivitis. Although variations in the calibre of the conjunctival vessels, with small microaneurysms or capillary dilation, may be found in the diabetic, such features are difficult to distinguish from inconsequential vascular anomalies also seen in the non-diabetic.

Eye muscles (see also diabetic mononeuropathies)

About one-third of isolated external ocular palsies prove to be diabetic. The sixth cranial nerve is most commonly involved, with partial third-nerve damage next in frequency. Combinations of these, or other external ocular muscles, are uncommon. The features of squint and diplopia usually recover within 3 to 4 months and recurrences are rare.

Anterior uvea

Rubeosis iridis is the name given to new vessel formation of the iris which usually develops in diabetic patients having advanced retinal disease. In diabetics, the lesion is usually bilateral, whereas in the non-diabetic, when the lesion is caused by a central retinal vein occlusion, it is unilateral. Rubeosis may not always be evident on naked eye examination and is best detected by careful slit-lamp observation. The disorder carries a poor prognosis because the patient is likely to develop secondary glaucoma, and the abnormal vessels may bleed excessively if surgery is undertaken.

Lens opacities

In general, diabetics are liable to develop simple senile cataracts about 10 to 15 years earlier than in non-diabetics. It is always a wise precaution to exclude diabetes in the case of any patient presenting with cataract. In the elderly diabetic, cataracts are of the ordinary senile variety, being either cortical or nuclear or a combination of both.

Young insulin-dependent diabetics may rarely develop a rapidly progressive form of lens opacity. The opacity starts with granularity of the central or posterior part of the nucleus and rapidly progresses. The vision deteriorates severely over a few months, although improved control of the diabetes can sometimes arrest or even reverse the process.

Intra-ocular tension and glaucoma

The majority of diabetic patients are in the older age group in which chronic simple glaucoma is common. Thus, even if there is no evidence of rubeosis iridis, the intra-ocular tension should be checked before dilating the pupil to examine the optic fundi.

Diabetic retinopathy

The fundamental elements of diabetic retinopathy are:
Microaneurysms and small blot haemorrhages are seen through the ophthalmoscope as discrete small round red areas. Examination of the capillary bed by fluorescein angiography has demonstrated that microaneurysms arise from alteration in capillary flow and redistribution consequent upon capillary closure. Microaneurysms usually start on the venous side of the capillary bed before extending to involve the arterial side. Blot haemorrhages are slightly larger variants, which are held in shape by the connective tissue fibres of the deeper layers of the retina.
Venous dilatation: This is also an early feature of diabetic retinopathy. As capillary closure progresses, however, areas of marked venous irregularity may develop, with small sausage-like dilatations appearing along the veins, which are thereafter at risk of haemorrhage. Marked

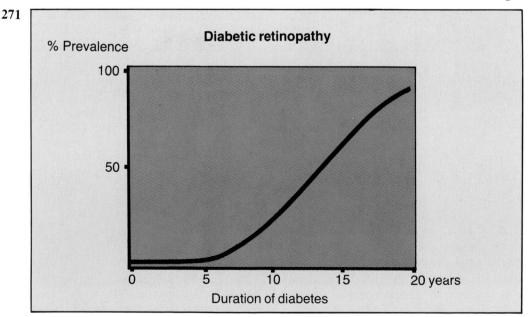

271

271 Prevalence of diabetic retinopathy. Rarely evident at diagnosis in the juvenile-onset diabetic. After 20 years duration the majority of these patients have evidence of retinal disease.

unilateral venous dilatation, however, may result from a venous occlusion rather than diabetic retinopathy.

Haemorrhage: These may be either blot haemorrhages in areas of microaneurysms or capillary closure; or larger flame-shaped lesions close to the surface of the retina and free from the constraints of connective tissue. They may also spread as linear streaks with an upper level affected by gravity.

Hard exudates: Hard exudates represent areas of lipid infiltration as a consequence of leakage from capillaries, although they may also result from local damage to neuronal tissue which has a high lipid content. They vary in shape and size according to whether the exudates are new small areas of leakage or have coalesced over a period of months or years. Hard exudates, which tend to have a yellowish colour, can be found anywhere in the retina, although they tend to be concentrated in the posterior pole where they coalesce into ring forms. The lesions have little effect upon vision unless they cover the fovea.

Cotton wool spots have a fluffy greyish-white appearance with indistinct edges and represent small areas of retinal ischaemia in an active phase. They have prognostic significance because their presence is a warning that the retinopathy may proceed to new vessel formation.

Neovascularisation: This is the main danger signal of diabetic retinopathy. New vessels may form either flat on the retina or protrude into the vitreous, sometimes surrounded by a sheath of fibrous tissue. The pathogenesis of new vessel formation relates to local retinal hypoxia; this hypoxia is consequent upon pre-capillary arteriolar insufficiency with focal capillary closure. These lesions are most likely to develop in diabetics having other evidence of underlying circulatory defects such as microaneurysms or cotton wool spots.

Vitreous: Abnormal new vessels may extend forward into the vitreous, forming a vascular network like seaweed floating in a rock pool (rete mirabile). Bleeding from new vessels causes vitreous haemorrhage and this is the commonest cause of sudden deterioration in vision in a diabetic known to have retinopathy. These haemorrhages clear spontaneously but are prone to recur. Repeated haemorrhages stimulate a fibrous reaction in the vitreous and further new vessel formation. The more severe fibrous reactions eventually contract and cause retinal detachment. Sometimes a large haemorrhage will cause complete opacity of the vitreous with total loss of vision.

Diabetic retinopathy can be classified into the following clinical groups, according to the nature and extent of the above elements.

Background retinopathy

This term applies to the earlier stages of retinal disease when scattered microaneurysms, venous dilatation or irregularity, and a few hard exudates are visible, but more ominous features such as new vessels, vitreous haemorrhage or fibrous tissue are not evident. At this stage visual acuity may be unaffected. Repeated examination will often confirm that microaneurysms can come and go. Nevertheless, the tendency is for these lesions to increase in number and extent over the course of a few years. Simple background retinopathy is the expected finding after 15 to 20 years of insulin-dependent diabetes. On the other hand, in maturity-onset diabetes, 10 per cent of patients will reveal background retinopathy at the time of diagnosis.

Maculopathy

This results from an extension of background retinopathy in which large plaques of hard exudate develop particularly above, below and lateral to the macula. Microaneurysms, blot or more superficial haemorrhages may also be evident and, although difficult to detect except by the experienced ophthalmologist, considerable macular oedema may be present. Both oedema and the presence of exudates in the region of the fovea can cause significant reduction in central vision. Characteristically, maculopathy affects late-onset diabetics, though it may also develop as a complication of background retinopathy in the long-standing insulin-dependent diabetic. Because detection of macular oedema is difficult with an ophthalmoscope, accurate assessment requires either binocular slit-lamp examination or fluorescein angiography.

Proliferative retinopathy

New vessel formation (neovascularisation) may develop slowly in an eye where background retinopathy has been evident for a few years; this usually responds well to light coagulation therapy. Much less commonly, a rapidly progressive florid form may occur with little evidence of previous retinal involvement. This florid form requires more extensive and urgent coagulation, if vitreous haemorrhage is to be avoided. Generally, however, treatment is less successful.

Careful examination through a dilated pupil is essential to exclude early evidence of new vessel formation, because at this stage the lesions are usually flat on the retinal surface, often well out in the periphery and unassociated with any visual defect.

Retinitis proliferans

Following the growth of new vessels into the vitreous, or vitreous haemorrhage, there is a second phase of growth of collagen and fibrous tissue, so that delicate vascular fronds become supported by a progressively dense network of connective tissues (retinitis proliferans). In almost half of the cases, the new vessels grow from the disc or from a major retinal vein. Generally, new vessels growing from the disc carry the worst prognosis in terms of developing retinitis proliferans. The more fibrous the tissue that develops, the greater the risk of contraction and retinal detachment.

Blindness and visual prognosis

Assessment of visual prognosis is complicated by the fact that sometimes even proliferative retinopathy undergoes spontaneous resolution. Early application of light coagulation has, however, reduced the rate and extent of visual deterioration. The five-year blindness rate for patients with untreated proliferative retinopathy is about 60 per cent. Pregnancy may worsen proliferative retinopathy. Thirty per cent of patients with untreated proliferative retinopathy who have a vitreous haemorrhage become blind in that eye within a year. If, however, vision survives longer than one year, then only a further 10 per cent become blind in the subsequent 3 years.

When one eye has been blinded by diabetic retinopathy, the prognosis for vision for the other eye is poor, unless treatment is undertaken promptly.

The prognosis for life in those blinded by proliferative retinopathy is less than 5 years on average, because of the almost invariable co-existence of renal or other vascular damage.

272

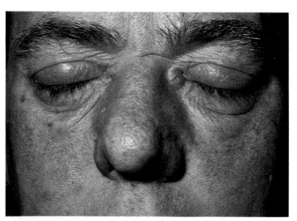

272 Blepharitis: inflammation and swelling of both upper and lower lids with encrusted eyelashes. This 56-year-old patient with a history of recurrent styes, was found to have glycosuria and hyperglycaemia at an eye clinic.

273

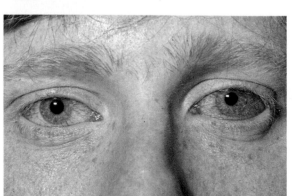

273 Severe conjunctivitis, which is common in diabetes.

274 Rubeosis iridis. A painful condition which sometimes develops in the diabetic with advanced retinal disease. New vessels form on the iris. There is associated oedema and high risk of secondary glaucoma.

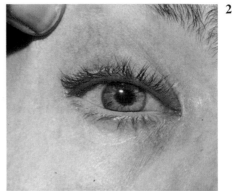

275 Rubeosis iridis: slit-lamp examination showing extensive new vessel formation in a diabetic patient with advanced retinal disease, who also developed secondary glaucoma.

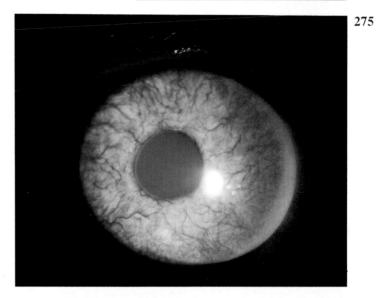

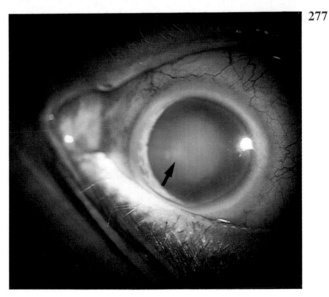

276 Rubeosis iridis showing marked new vessel formation in one section of the iris (arrowed) on slit-lamp examination.

277 Nuclear cataract demonstrated by slit-lamp examination showing dense grey opacification of nuclear portion of lens.

113

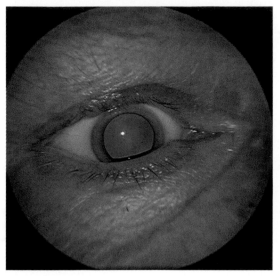

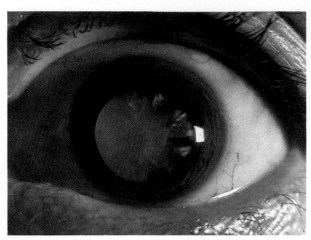

27

279 Senile cataract. This occurs at a younger age in diabetes than in other patients.

278 Clear normal lens in comparison with **277**.

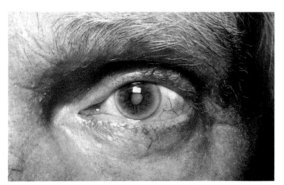

280 Senile cataract: grey opacity of lens and arcus senilis in a 65-year-old maturity-onset diabetic.

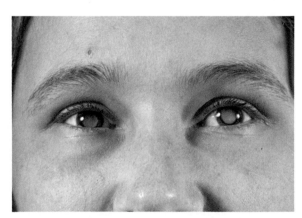

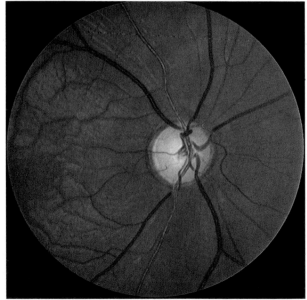

28

281 Juvenile type cataract in a 20-year-old girl with diabetes of 15 years duration. Rapidly progressive granular opacities developed in the lenses some 2 years previously, when the diabetes was poorly controlled.

282 Congenital optic atrophy associated with diabetes. A rare genetic disorder which may be part of the DIDMOAD (Diabetes insipidus, diabetes mellitus, optic atrophy, deafness) syndrome (see Chapter 2).

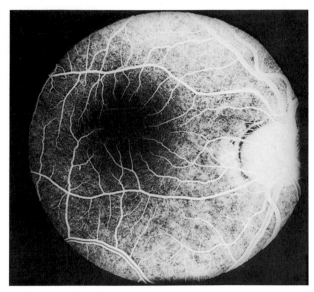

283 Normal fundus. Fluorescein is injected intravenously and retinal photographs are taken in rapid sequence in the arterial phase, revealing the circulation in the retinal capillary bed. (*Fluorescein angiogram*)

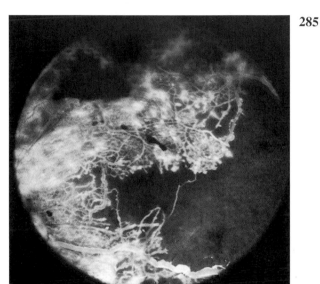

284 Blindness in a 20-year-old diabetic girl after 17 years of diabetes.

285 Widespread capillary microaneurysms revealed in a fluorescein angiogram.

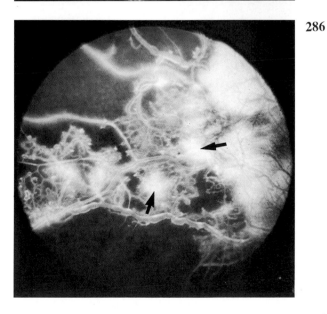

286 Extensive capillary leakage due to breakdown of the capillary-retinal barrier. Fluorescein angiogram at a later phase.

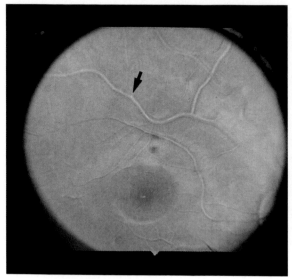

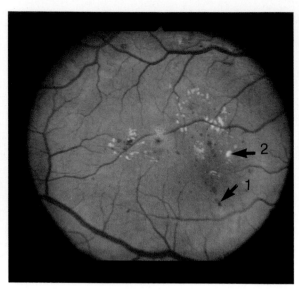

287 Lipaemia retinalis associated with severe hyperlipidaemia in controlled diabetes (see page 86). The very high plasma lipid content makes the plasma milky and the retinal vessels appear white.

288 Early background retinopathy showing scattered microaneurysms (1) and hard exudates (2).

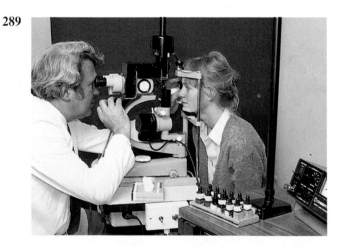

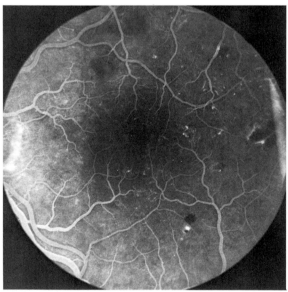

289 Photocoagulation for diabetic retinopathy using the argon laser. Destruction of new vessel formation by photocoagulation prevents deterioration from haemorrhages.

290 Early background retinopathy. Only one microaneurysm was seen at ophthalmoscopy, but many more are visible on fluorescein examination indicating the value of this technique in assessing the extent of retinal disease.

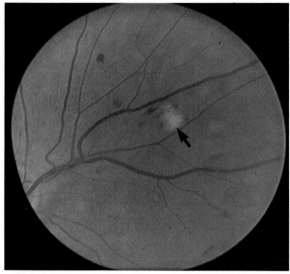

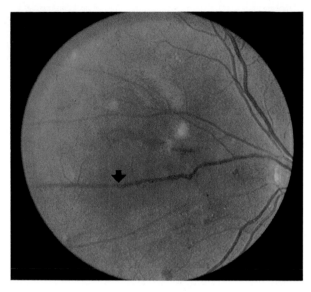

291 Background retinopathy in a diabetic showing a cotton wool spot in the centre of the field (arrowed). These are areas of retinal infarction and evidence of deterioration in the retinal microcirculation.

292 Venous irregularity. A vein running horizontally across the retina (arrowed) showing marked 'beading' in a patient with background retinopathy. There are several cotton wool spots, microaneurysms and blot haemorrhages in the same field. Venous irregularity may be followed by haemorrhage into the vitreous.

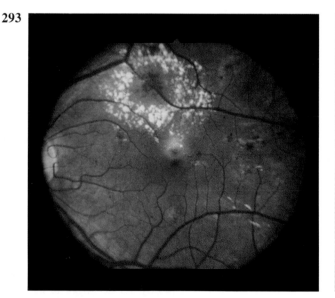

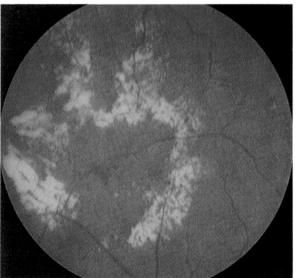

293 Predominantly exudative retinopathy. The hard exudates encompass the fovea in a circinate formation. Macular oedema is present. The combination of hard exudates and oedema (known as diabetic maculopathy) can cause significant loss of vision.

294 Extensive circinate hard exudates and oedema with resultant maculopathy and visual deterioration.

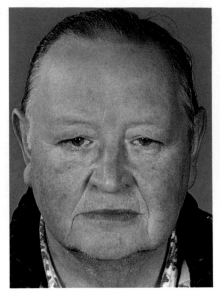

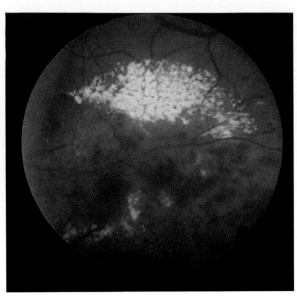

295 Maturity-onset diabetic newly diagnosed, presenting to optician with blurred vision.

296 Extensive retinal exudative retinopathy already present in the same patient (**295**) at diagnosis.

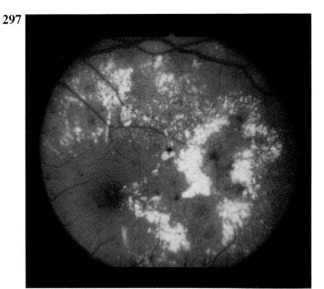

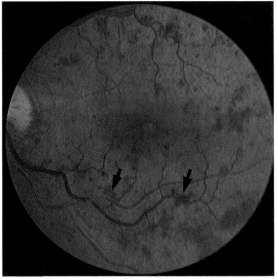

297 Extensive exudation in an elderly mild diabetic. Despite the extent of the lesions the macula was not involved, so that there was only moderate deterioration in reading vision.

298 Venous thrombosis in a diabetic. Although similar to the lesion in non-diabetics, it occurs more commonly in diabetics and may be unassociated with other features of diabetic retinal disease. Capillary engorgement and haemorrhage along the whole length of vessel and unilateral lesion are clues to the diagnosis.

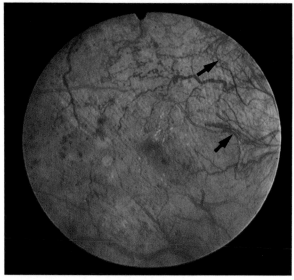

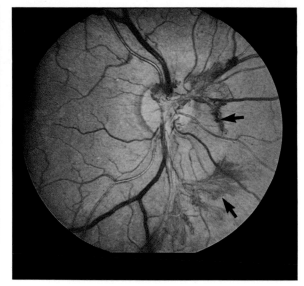

299 **Proliferative retinopathy:** numerous small new vessels (neovascularisation) throughout the retina.

300 **Proliferative retinopathy.** Fronds of new vessels emerging from the disc and elsewhere.

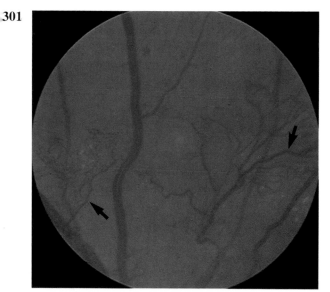

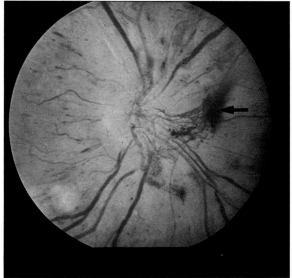

301 **Neovascular tissue** before visible leakage or haemorrhage has occurred.

302 **Proliferative retinopathy.** New vessels may grow forwards into the vitreous leading to haemorrhage in the retina and into the vitreous. The arrow indicates a small pre-retinal haemorrhage.

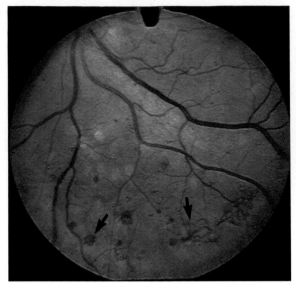

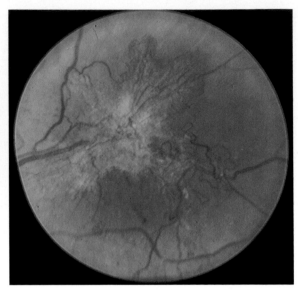

303 Proliferative retinopathy. Network of friable new vessels with numerous small haemorrhages.

304 Advanced neovascularisation. Fronds of new vessels with fibrous tissue protruding into the vitreous.

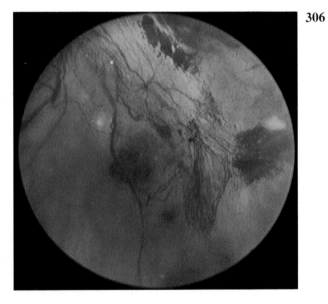

305 Proliferative retinopathy. Neovascularisation leading to extensive gliosis (fibrosis—arrowed) of the retina. Serious loss of vision inevitably ensues, often from retinal detachment.

306 Vitreous haze due to bleeding from several areas of new vessels, with fibrous tissue in the background.

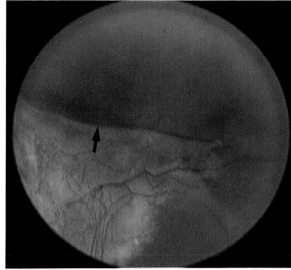

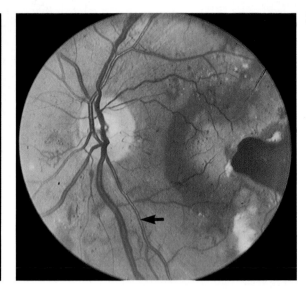

307 **Vitreous haze** in the upper half of the field showing horizontal lower level (arrowed) which might be mistaken for a blood vessel. Extensive fibrosis and neovascularisation is seen in the remainder of the field. Loss of vision and risk of retinal detachment is present by contracting fibrous tissue.

308 **Macular subhyaloid pre-retinal haemorrhage** in a hypertensive diabetic. Note reactive hypertensive sclerosis (silver-wiring) in retinal arterioles (arrowed). Hypertension adds to the risk of haemorrhage in diabetic retinopathy. This diabetic had no further bleeding after control of the hypertension.

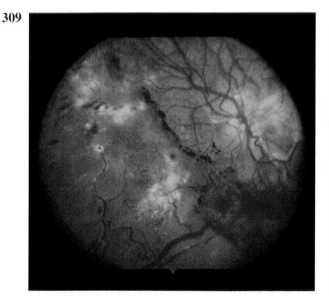

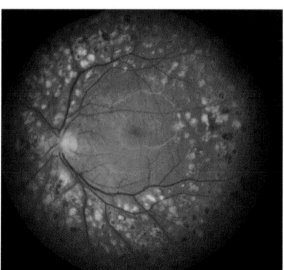

309 **Proliferative retinopathy and maculopathy.** Neovascularisation with free haemorrhage. Venous dilatation and macular oedema.

310 **Argon laser photocoagulation** for treatment of proliferative diabetic retinopathy has resulted in numerous pigmented scars in the peripheral retina. Dark adaptation may be affected.

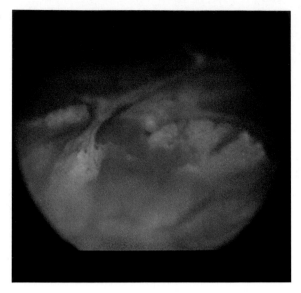

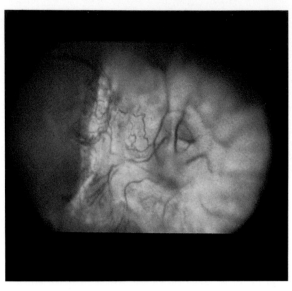

311 Retinitis proliferans with severe gliosis and vitreous detachment. Perception of light only.

312 Retinitis proliferans. Total destruction of the retina by extensive gliosis.

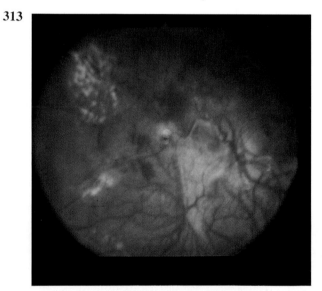

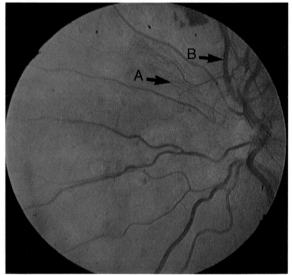

313 Continuing vitreous haemorrhage, fibrosis and new vessel formation.

314 Fine new vessels (A) and dilated veins (B) both of which are at risk of haemorrhage. Prophylactic treatment with photocoagulation considerably reduces the dangers in this situation.

315
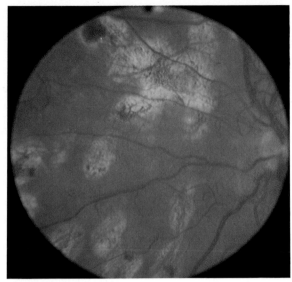

316
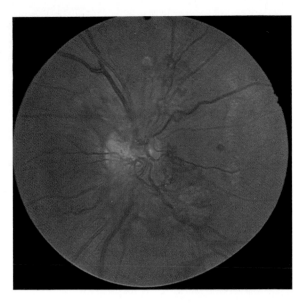

315 **After treatment** with xenon arc photocoagulation (arrowed) in the same patient (313).

316 **Widespread new vessels** including new vessels arising from the disc. The proximity of the vessels to the disc makes photocoagulation difficult.

317
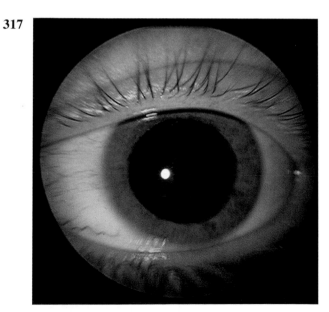

317 **Sudden loss of vision** after extensive vitreous haemorrhage. Loss of light reflex (dilated pupil).

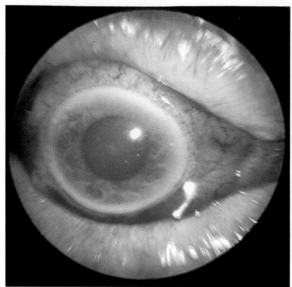

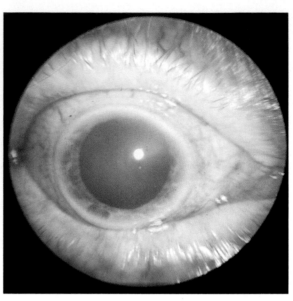

318   Blood in vitreous following extensive hae-morrhage in a diabetic known to have prolifera-tive retinopathy. Treated by intravitreal injection units of urokinase.

319   Clearing of the vitreous in the same patient (317) 15 days later. Useful vision returned.

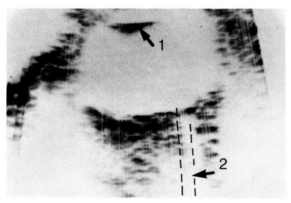

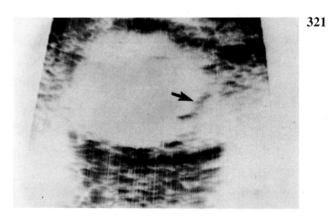

320   B-scan ultrasound of an eye in a patient with advanced vitreous haemorrhage similar to 317. No evidence of fibrous reaction at this level. (1 = lens, 2 = optic nerve.)

321   B-scan ultrasound at a different level from 320 showing a small band of 'fibrous' reaction (arrow). This examination is a useful guide to the ophthalmologist in cases of advanced haemorr-hage, because extensive fibrous reaction is unlikely to respond to urokinase.

11 The kidney and lower renal tract

Renal damage in diabetes mellitus is a slow and insidious process which is often overlooked. Its progress and development closely parallel the course of diabetic retinopathy but, whereas retinopathy is readily detected with the ophthalmoscope, renal involvement may be much more difficult to diagnose without percutaneous biopsy.

'Diabetic nephropathy' is a useful general term embracing the various glomerular, arteriolar and infective lesions which can occur in the diabetic kidney. To understand the clinical development of renal failure, several steps in a complicated process have to be considered. The disorder starts with a metabolic change in the structure of the basement membrane ground substance of the glomerular capillaries, which becomes thicker and more porous. Mesangial expansion takes place at the same time. The filtration properties of the glomerulus become modified, leading to proteinuria and fibrin deposition within the glomerular capillaries. Haemodynamic changes lead to arteriolar damage and a characteristic nodular lesion within the glomerulus, which was first described by Kimmelstiel and Wilson in 1936. As a consequence of the glomerular capillary and arteriolar lesions, the kidney becomes increasingly ischaemic and simultaneously more susceptible to infection—ascending pyelonephritis or, more rarely, renal papillary necrosis.

Basement membrane thickening

The fine structure of the glomerulus can be seen in clear detail with the electron microscope. This shows the homogeneous basement membrane of the capillary wall bounded by epithelial foot processes and endothelial cytoplasm. The characteristic change in diabetes is a gradual and sustained increase in basement membrane material, leading to diffuse thickening of the capillary wall and accumulation of basement membrane in the capillary stalk or mesangium. Unlike non-diabetic renal disease, the epithelial cytoplasm which is responsible for basement membrane synthesis is well preserved. Normally, basement membrane is an amorphous collagen-like glycoprotein containing 10 per cent of carbohydrate. In hyperglycaemia, the glycopro-

tein structure is modified as a consequence of the increased incorporation of carbohydrate and the simultaneous diminution in amino-acid cross-linkages. This abnormal configuration of the thickened glycoprotein basement membrane increases permeability to plasma proteins and other macromolecules.

Normal basement membrane turnover is a combination of epithelial synthesis and removal by the mesangial cells. Basement membrane accumulation in diabetes may be further increased by loss of mesangial cell function.

Altered membrane permeability leads to the deposition of fibrin within the capillary wall and mesangial stalk, leading to the development of various small blood vessel lesions which can be seen on light microscopy of either renal biopsy or autopsy tissue.

Light microscopy of renal biopsy or autopsy tissue

Glomerular lesions

Types of glomerular lesions are as follows: diffuse; nodular Kimmelstiel-Wilson lesion; exudate; and hyalinisation. 'Diabetic glomerulosclerosis' is the general term for these lesions, which often co-exist. Their common end point is glomerular hyalinisation.

Diffuse glomerular lesion
The severity of renal failure and nephrotic syndrome correlate best with this glomerular lesion, which is the commonest finding in the diabetic kidney. The lesion is not, however, pathognomonic because other non-diabetic forms of diffuse glomerulosclerosis cannot be distinguished from the diabetic lesion without electron microscopy.

Nodular glomerular lesion
Although less common than the diffuse lesion, the nodule is regarded as diagnostic of diabetes by the light microscopist. Within an affected glomerulus, which may be normal in size or slightly enlarged, nodules occupy the centres of single or multiple

lobules. The fully developed lesion may be an almost spherical, homogeneous, vacuolated fibrillar or lamellar mass, often having a patent or distended capillary running over its surface. The main diagnostic features are: the nodule is focal, peripheral, centrilobular and acellular.

Exudative glomerular lesion

The exudative lesion is the least specific of the glomerular changes in diabetes, occurring also in various non-diabetic glomerular disorders associated with renal failure. The lesion usually consists of rounded or crescentic deposits of either homogeneous or vacuolated, intensely acidophilic material without nuclei, representing various proteins and fibrinoid which have leaked into the glomerular lumen.

Glomerular hyalinisation

As a consequence of the above lesions, increasing numbers of glomeruli become completely hyalinised in advanced cases. There may be shrinkage of the glomerular tuft or peri-glomerular fibrosis, with thickening of the Bowman's capsule by connective tissue fibrils.

Tubular lesions

Various lesions may be found in the tubules of diabetics, few are of specific significance and in general they are secondary to glomerulosclerosis, ischaemia, pyelonephritis or longstanding electrolyte disturbance.

The 'Armanni-Ebstein lesion', or 'glycogen nephrosis', first described in 1877, consists of glycogen-laden vacuoles in the tubules of the corticomedullary region. A common post-mortem finding in the pre-insulin era, this is now occasionally found in those who die following uncorrected hyperglycaemia, acidosis and dehydration.

Arteriolar lesions

Hyaline lesions affect both the afferent and efferent arterioles in diabetes. Although similar to the fibrinoid lesion of the hypertensive kidney, normotensic diabetics often have more marked arteriolar disease than hypertensive patients.

Interstitial tissue

Urinary tract infections

Several factors may predispose the diabetic to urinary tract infection. Diabetic autonomic neuropathy favours bladder stasis; catheterisation when the patient is in coma may introduce sepsis and infection is more likely in renal tissue affected by arteriosclerosis and glomerulosclerosis. The pathologist bases a diagnosis of infection on histological features, which include lymphocytic infiltration of the intertubular tissue, periglomerular fibrosis and increased connective tissue. Because these changes could result from either ischaemia or chronic pyelonephritis, the histological diagnosis is often difficult.

Tuberculosis

When tuberculosis was more common in the western world, there was an apparent excess of the disease in diabetics, perhaps because these patients attended hospital regularly and had a better chance of diagnosis. Nevertheless, tuberculosis should always be excluded when chronic renal infection is suspected and regular chest radiology is still a wise precaution for diabetics. Although active pulmonary and renal tubercle do not usually co-exist, the finding of either old healed pulmonary tubercle, or of a tuberculoma are pointers to the possibility that chronic renal infection may be tuberculous. A tuberculoma is a more common finding in diabetics and may not be confined to the upper lobes of the lungs. This can make it radiologically difficult to exclude the alternative of lung cancer or an isolated secondary from renal or other neoplasia.

Renal papillary necrosis

This is usually initiated by acute infection in which the tips of the medullary tissue become necrotic. In the diabetic the lesion may be exacerbated by ischaemia leading to sloughing of papillae with profuse haematuria and ureteric obstruction. With improved antibiotic therapy, one of the main causes of papillary necrosis today is the abuse of analgesics rather than infection.

Evolution of diabetic nephropathy

There is no reliable evidence that glomerular capillary basement membrane lesions ever precede the onset of juvenile diabetes. The initial progress of the ultrastructural defects is slow. Even after 20 years of insulin-dependent diabetes the basement membrane may be only slightly more than double its normal thickness, although at this stage diffuse glomerulosclerosis will be evident on light microscopy.

As basement membrane and fibrin accumulate in the mesangium, the mesangial area enlarges, thus reducing the vascular and urinary space within the glomerulus. Adverse haemodynamic consequences then follow and cause occlusion of peripheral lobules and nodule formation. Many of the features in the interstitial tissue which resemble healed chronic pyelonephritis may be secondary to ischaemia; nevertheless, the diabetic kidney is particularly vulnerable to infection in the later stages of the disease.

Clinical features

The main clinical features are as follows: proteinuria; peripheral oedema; renal failure; normochronic anaemia; hypertension; and pyelonephritis.

None of these is specific to diabetes; patients are often found to have advanced renal disease (either at renal biopsy or at post-mortem) without clinical features having been evident. The patient's vitality is sapped away and yet chronic deterioration in kidney function may be difficult to detect.

Proteinuria
Although generally regarded as the classic sign of diabetic nephropathy, effective monitoring of filtered protein by the healthy glomerular epithelium may diminish excretion in the early stages, so that assessment on the basis of proteinuria may be unrealistic. Nevertheless, the presence of proteinuria constitutes reasonably reliable evidence of diabetic glomerulosclerosis, provided that cardiac failure, pyuria or ketoacidosis are excluded. In patients over 60 years of age, proteinuria is most common due to cardiac failure. Because proteinuria is often initially intermittent, a 24-hour urine collection for total protein estimation is the best guide to severity. Tests of differential protein clearance do not clarify the diagnosis.

Oedema
This is often due to other causes. For example, oedema sometimes occurs temporarily after insulin therapy is introduced or increased. Oedema in diabetes may be due to cardiac disease. Oedema in diabetic glomerulosclerosis is most marked at the stage when glomeruli are diffusely affected before hyalinisation develops. At this stage proteinuria may be in the region of 6g per 24 hours and the blood urea only marginally elevated.

Renal failure
The glomerular filtration rate falls with increasing histological abnormality: serum creatinine should be determined regularly in all patients with proteinuria. Changes of the inverse of the creatinine approximately reflect those of the GFR (glomerular filtration rate) which is difficult to assess in routine clinical practice.

Anaemia
Normochronic and normocytic anaemia—mainly due to failure of erythropoiesis—is common and is unresponsive to haematinics. Iron and folate deficiency should be excluded, however, especially if the patient's diet plan is protein restricted.

Hypertension
Hypertension plays an important role in the development and progression of diabetic nephropathy, although often renal arteriolar lesions may precede hypertension. Patients with a family history of hypertension may be more likely to develop nephropathy. Vigorous treatment of hypertension may slow the progression of the disease.

Pyelonephritis
Diabetic nephropathy and autonomic neuropathy may be the underlying causes of this disorder, particularly when found in males.

Diagnosis

Because the clinical features of diabetic nephropathy are essentially non-specific, accurate diagnosis depends upon percutaneous renal biopsy. This is not usually required, and if specific diabetic retinopathy is evident, diabetic nephropathy is an almost certain accompaniment.

Prevalence
Assessment is difficult without reliable diagnostic methods. Long duration of juvenile-onset insulin-dependent diabetes is the most important factor. After 20 years duration, some degree of nephropathy will be evident at biopsy, whereas in late-onset diabetes, nephropathy may be present at diagnosis or appear within a few years.

Prognosis
Patients who present with clinical features of diabetic nephropathy—or histological evidence at biopsy of Kimmelstiel-Wilson nodules, exudative lesions or glomerular hyalinisation—have a poor prognosis. In the early stages, improved diabetic control may reverse microproteinuria and it is important to treat hypertension effectively, often with ACE (angiotensin converting enzyme) inhibitors, which diminish efferent glomerular arteriolar spasm. The outlook will also be affected by the presence or absence of other specific or non-specific complications. In established uraemia, death may often result from some other vascular episode. Kidney transplants must be considered at an earlier stage and may be life-saving; it may be best performed when the serum creatinine is between 400 and 600 mmol/l.

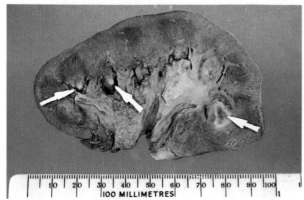

322 Necrosis of renal papillae (arrowed) is occasionally a feature of diabetic nephropathy.

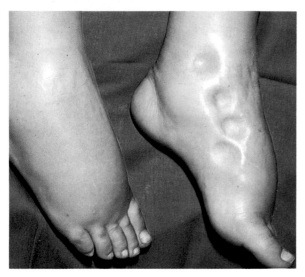

323 Gross pitting oedema after 20 years insulin-dependent diabetes. Heavy proteinuria (6g per 24 hours). Slightly elevated blood urea (10mmol/litre). Blood pressure 180/100mmHg. Clinical diagnosis of diabetic nephropathy confirmed by percutaneous renal biopsy (**324**).

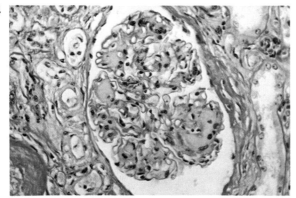

324 Glomerulus from 323 showing diffuse and nodular glomerulosclerosis. Generalised thickening of capillary walls throughout the glomerular lobules.

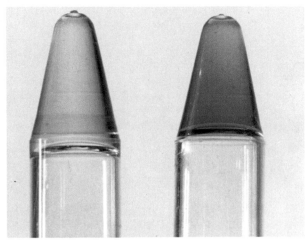

325 Quantifying macroproteinuria in diabetic nephropathy. Two urine specimens are diluted and reacted with a protein-building dye. After precipitation and re-dissolving, the dye-bound protein is quantitated spectrophotometrically. The specimen on the left originally contained 10g protein/1; the one on the right contained no detectable protein.

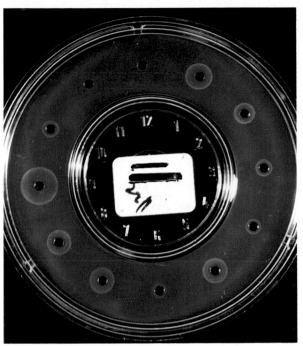

326 Detection of trace amount of albumin in urine by radial immunodiffusion (RID). The specimens are placed in the wells shown and diffuse into the surrounding gel which contains anti-albumin antiserum. The concentration of albumin in the sample is proportional to the diameter of the precipitation ring formed. In this illustration, wells 1-4 are standard ones.

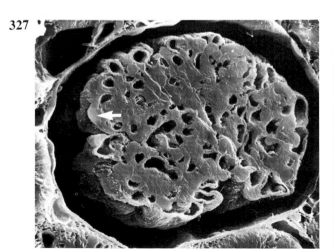

327 Diabetic rat glomerulus showing diffuse thickening of capillary walls (arrowed) similar to human diabetic glomerulosclerosis (see **324**). (*Scanning electron micrograph* × *600*)

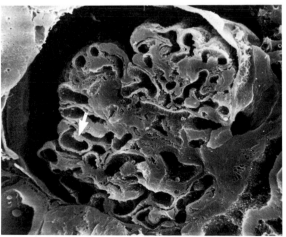

328 Non-diabetic rat glomerulus for comparison with **329**. Note the thin capillary walls and more open capillary loops (arrowed). (*Scanning electron micrograph* × *600*)

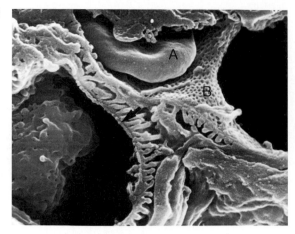

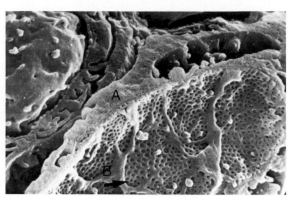

330 Diabetic rat glomerulus showing a thickened basement membrane (A) and pores (B) in the endothelial cytoplasm. (*Scanning electron micrograph × 5 000*)

329 Non-diabetic rat glomerulus showing thin basement membrane (arrowed), a red blood cell (A) with a capillary loop and pores in the endothelial cytoplasm (B). (*Scanning electron micrograph × 5 000*)

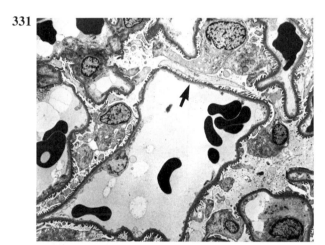

331 Glomerular capillary loops in juvenile-onset insulin-dependent diabetic of 2 years' duration. No evidence of capillary basement membrane thickening (arrowed). Note dilated capillary loop, which is associated with the increased glomerular filtration rate of early diabetes. (*Electron micrograph × 1 000*)

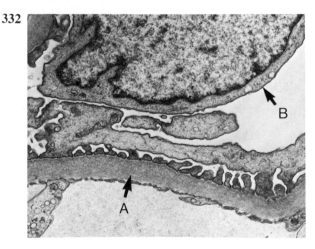

332 Glomerular capillary basement membrane thickening. Electron micrograph of biopsy tissue from insulin-dependent diabetic of 15 years' duration, showing the characteristic homogeneous increase in basement membrane glycoprotein (A). Unlike other forms of non-diabetic glomerulosclerosis, the epithelium (B) and foot processes are well-preserved. (*× 10 000*)

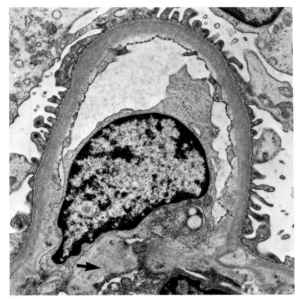

333 Glomerular capillary loop from case **331** showing basement membrane thickening and accumulation of basement membrane material in capillary stalk or mesangium (arrowed).(× *8 000*)

335 Glomerular lobule from **331** showing more extensive replacement of mesangium, with basement membrane material (A)—the forerunner of the Kimmelstiel-Wilson nodule. (× *2 000*)

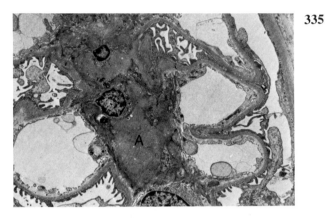

334 Basement membrane accumulating in mesangium (arrowed) in **331** and encroaching upon mesangial cell cytoplasm. (× *5 000*)

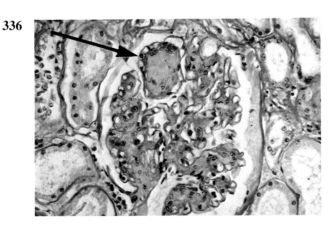

336 Diffuse glomerulosclerosis and early Kimmelstiel-Wilson nodules (arrowed) in light microscopy of glomerulus. (*MSB × 250*)

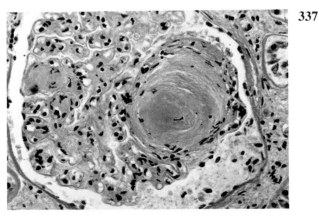

337 The Kimmelstiel-Wilson nodule. Glomerulus from autopsy on longstanding diabetic showing a characteristic large, acellular, peripheral nodule on a background of diffuse diabetic glomerulosclerosis. (*MSB × 250*)

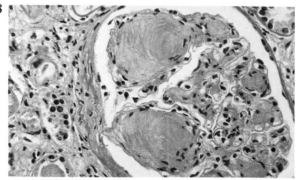

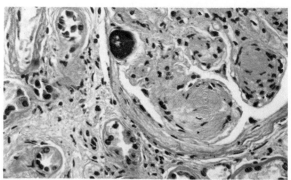

338 Multiple Kimmelstiel-Wilson nodules in another glomerulus from **336**. This finding in an unknown diabetic would allow the pathologist to make a confident histological diagnosis of diabetes mellitus. (*MSB × 250*)

339 Diffuse and nodular glomerulosclerosis with small red-staining fibrinoid lesion—exudative glomerulosclerosis, from **338**. (*MSB × 250*)

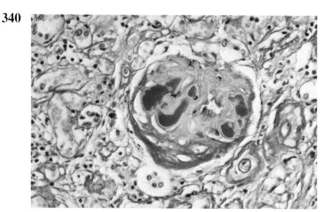

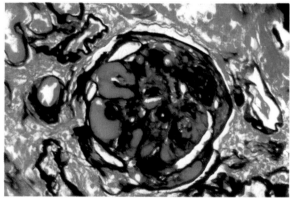

340 Exudative glomerulosclerosis. Multiple scarlet-staining fibrinoid lesions, which may also occur in non-diabetic forms of glomerular damage. Found at autopsy on a longstanding diabetic who died in renal failure. (*MSB × 200*)

341 Glomerulus from **339** showing extensive dark stain for basement membrane material characteristic of diabetes.(*Silver × 200*)

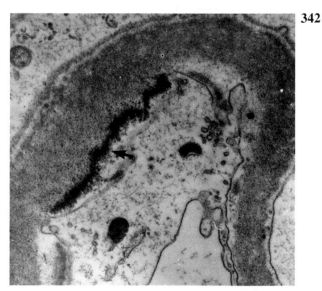

342 Band of fibrin-derived macromolecules along the border of capillary basement membrane from a patient without evidence of fibrin on MSB staining. Fibrin is probably laid down at an early stage as a consequence of altered glomerular permeability.(*Electron micrograph × 20 000*)

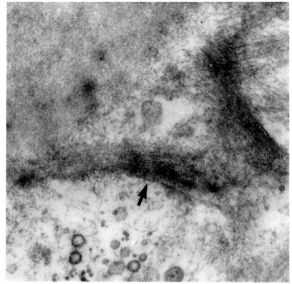

343 Linear bundles of early fibrin being laid down alongside glomerular capillary basement membrane.(*Electron micrograph × 40 000*)

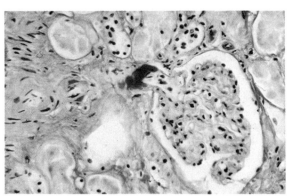

344 Arteriolar lesion in diabetes. Scarlet-staining fibrinoid lesion in afferent arteriole. Similar to lesion seen in hypertension, but commonly found in normotensive diabetics who tend to develop both afferent and efferent arteriosclerosis.(*MSB × 150*)

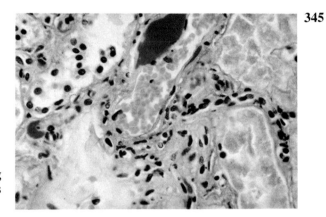

345 Arteriolar lesion showing scarlet-staining fibrinoid material in vessel wall. Red blood cells stain yellow.(*MSB × 400*)

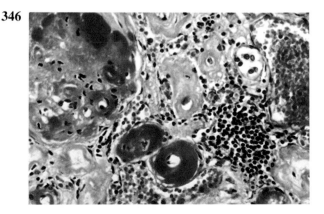

346 Afferent and efferent arteriosclerosis and glomerulosclerosis. H&E stain which does not allow discrimination between fibrinoid and hyaline material.(× 200)

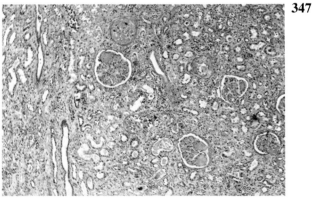

347 Low-power view showing various glomerular lesions with ischaemic changes and chronic inflammatory cells in the interstitial tissue. There is difficulty in distinguishing, on histological grounds, between ischaemia and chronic pyelonephritis. (*MSB × 50*)

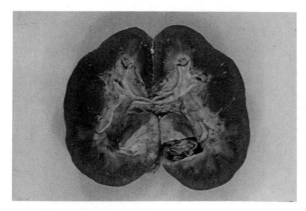

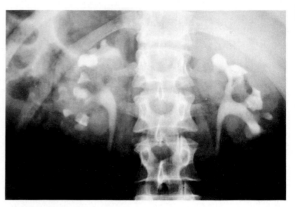

348 Post-mortem section of kidney with chronic pyelonephritis. Note irregularity of cortex and hydronephrosis.

349 Chronic pyelonephritis. IVP from 45-year-old diabetic showing bilateral clubbing of the calyces and patchy loss of cortical substance.

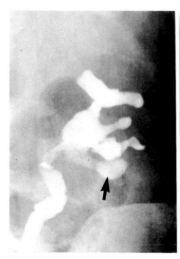

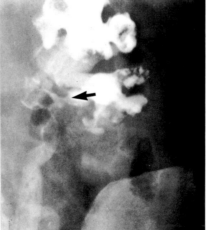

350 Renal papillary necrosis. Retrograde pyelogram showing (left) marked calyceal clubbing and distortion. One month later (right) sloughing of calyceal tissue into the renal pelvis is evident.

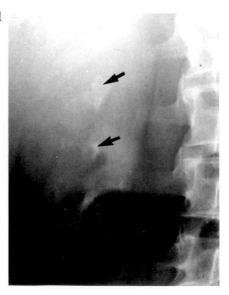

351 Renal papillary necrosis. IVP showing poor renal function and calyceal 'ring shadows' (arrowed) characteristic of papillary necrosis. With improved antibiotic therapy this is now a rare lesion in diabetes and is more commonly associated with analgesic abuse.

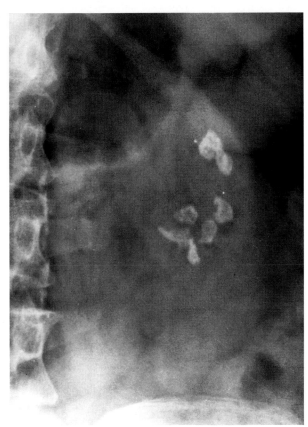

352 **Renal papillary necrosis** of longstanding showing calicification of papillae, which had sloughed some years previously.

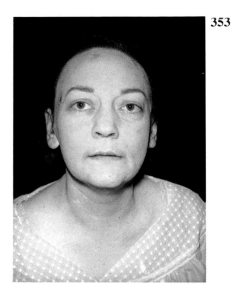

353 **Terminal uraemia in a diabetic woman.** Note pallor due to secondary normochromic and normocytic anaemia. She is totally blind and has severe neuropathy.

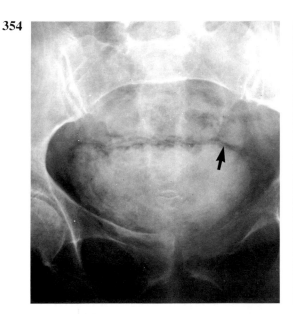

354 **Emphysematous cystitis.** Plain Xray showing gas tracking in the bladder wall. This is a 63-year-old diabetic female with clinical features of severe cystitis following treatment for carcinoma of the cervix.

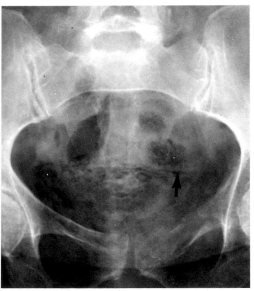

355 **IVP of the patient in 361** showing contrast in the bladder and again demonstrating gas outlining the irregular bladder wall (arrowed).

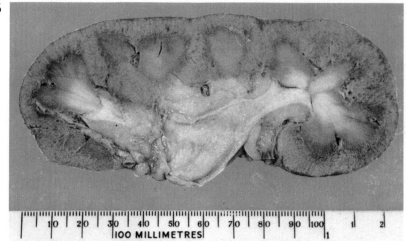

356 **Mild diabetic nephropathy.** Apart from pallor of some renal medullae there is no significant abnormality.

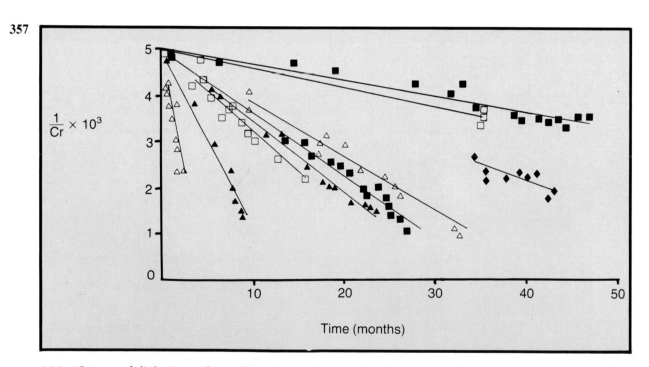

357 **Course of diabetic nephropathy** obtained by plotting the inverse of the serum cretinine umol/l against time: the decline of renal function is linear for each individual patient, but the rate of decline varies substantially from one patient to another.

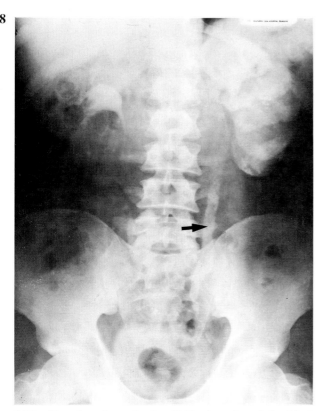

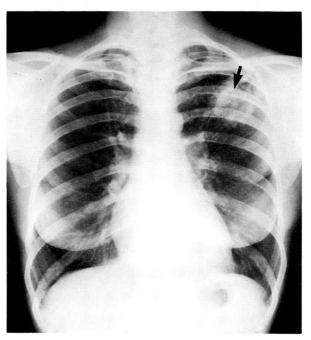

359 Pulmonary tuberculosis in a diabetic patient whose renal disease was thought to be tuberculous. Chest Xray showing a cavitating lesion in the left upper lobe with fibrosis and traction on the hilum. Renal biopsy showed that the kidney disease was diabetic in origin.

358 Renal tuberculosis. IVP showing left-sided hydronephrosis and hydro-ureter with extensive renal and ureteric calcification and dilatation of the ureter.

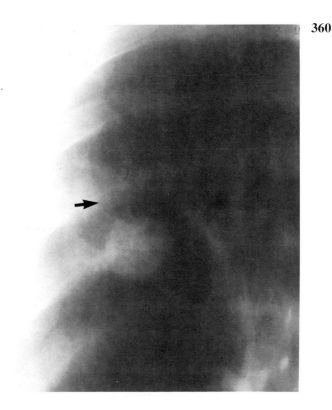

360 Tuberculoma in a diabetic. Tomogram showing coin lesion in the right midzone with ill-defined calcification. Chronic renal infection in this case was found to be tuberculous in origin.

Index

All numerals refer to page numbers

Diabetic Associations

Argentine League for the Protection
of Diabetics
Tucuman 1584
Buenos Aires, **Argentina**
Phone: 54-1/40 18 85

Argentinian Diabetes Society
Santa Fé 1171
(1059) Buenos Aires, **Argentina**
Telefax: 54-1/42 8419

Diabetes Australia
QBE Bldg., 33-35 Ainslie Ave.
Canberra A.C.T., P.O. Box 944
Civic Square A.C.T. 2608, **Australia**
Phone 1: 61-62/475655
Phone 2: 61-62/475722
Telefax: 61-62/573140

Austrian Diabetes Association
Moosstrasse 18
5020 Salzburg, **Austria,**
Phone: 43-222/82 09 753

Austrian Diabetes Society
c/o I. Medizinische Abteilung der
KA Rudolfstiftung
Juchgasse 25, A-1030 Wien, **Austria**
Phone: 43-222/71165/DW 400 od. 401

Diabetic Association of Bangladesh
Shahbagh Avenue
Dhaka 1000, **Bangladesh**
Phone 1: 880-2/40006-9
Phone 2: 880-2/404220
Telex: 642442 BPL BJ

Association Belge du Diabète
Chausée der Waterloo, 935
B-1180 Brussels, **Belgium**
Phone: 32-2/344 06 95

Belgian Association for Diabetics
BVS Secretariat
Charles de Kerchovelaan 369
B-9000 Ghent, **Belgium**
Phone: 32-91/20 05 20

Bermuda Diabetic Association
P.O. Box DV506
Devonshire, **Bermuda** DVBX
Phone: 1-809/292-1595

Brasilian Diabetes Society
Rua Conega José Loreto 9
Caneta
40140 Salvador, **Brazil**
Phone: 55-21/245 8555, 245 8156
Telefax: 55-21/245 1941

Brasilian Diabetes Association
Av. Paulista 2073
21 Andar-Sala 2123
Sao Paulo-CEP 01331, **Brazil**
Phone: 55-11/289-941

Bulgarian Society of Endocrinology
Inst. of Endocrinology and Gerontology
Christo Michailov Street 6
Sofia 1303, **Bulgaria**
Phone 1: 87 14 97
Phone 2: 87 72 01

Canadian Diabetes Association
78 Bond Street
Toronto, Ontario M5B 2J8, **Canada**
Phone: 1-416/362-4440
Telefax: 1-416/362-6849

L'Association du Diabète du Quebec
1160 rue Panet
Montreal, Quebec H2L 2Y7, **Canada**
Phone: 1-514/879 11 91

Chilean Society of Endocrinology and
Metabolism
Av. Presidente Riesco 6007
Las Condes
Santiago, **Chile**
Phone: 56-2/243175

Diabetes Section of the Chinese
Medical Association
42 Dongsi Xidajie
Beijing 100710, **China**
Phone 1: 55.0394
Phone 2: 55.7388

Colombian Diabetes Association
Calle 39A No. 14-78
Bogotá, **Colombia**
Phone 1: 57-2/885453
Phone 2: 57-2/885376

Costa Rican Association for
Endocrinology, Diabetes and Nutrition
Colegio de Medicos y Cirujanos
P.O. Box 548
1000 San Jose, **Costa Rica**
Phone: 506/323 433
Telex: 2149 AMES
Telefax: 506/322406

Cuban Diabetes Society
Consejo Cientifica
Edificio del Ministerio de Salud Publica
23 y N Vedado Habana 4, **Cuba**
Phone: 3-4971

Cyprus Diabetic Association
P.O. Box 302 Diana Court
Loizou Philippou St.
Paphos, **Cyprus**
Phone: 357-61/339 66

Czechoslovak Diabetology Association
Internal Clinic ILF
National Diabetes Program
Coordinating Center
762 75 Gottwaldov, **Czechoslovakia**
Phone: 42/28235
Telex: 672 00

Danish Diabetes Association
Filosofgangen 24
5000 Odense C, **Denmark**
Phone: 45-66/12 90 06
Telefax: 45-65/91 49 08

Dominican Diabetes Society
Apartado 1600
Santo Domingo, **Dominican Republic**

National Institute of Endocrinology
and Nutrition
P.O. Box 1600
Santo Domingo, **Dominican Republic**
Phone: 809/567-9251, 566-9693

Ecuadorian Diabetes Association
c/o Hospital Carlos Andrade Martin
Dept. Medico
Quito, **Ecuador**

Egyptian Union of Diabetic Associations
40, Safia Zaghloul St.
Alexandria, **Egypt**
Phone 1: 20-3/4822720
Phone 2: 20-3/844411

Ethiopian Diabetes Association
P.O. Box 31840
Addis Ababa, **Ethiopia**
Phone: 251-1/158174

Finnish Diabetes Association
Diabeteskeskus
SF-33680 Tampere, **Finland**
Phone: 358-31/600 333
Telefax: 358-31/600 462

Association Française des Diabétiques
14 rue du Clos
75020 Paris, **France**
Phone: 33-1/40 09 24 25
Telefax: 33-1/40 09 20 30

German Diabetes Union
Danzigerweg 1
D-5880 Lüdenscheid, **Germany**
Phone: 49-2351/85053

Ghana Diabetic Association
P.O. Box Korle-Bu
Accra, **Ghana**
Phone: 233/655401 Ext. 520

Hellenic Diabetologic Association
Papadiamandopoulou Street 4
GR-11528 Athens, **Greece**
Phone: 30-1/711 845

Panhellenic Diabetic Association
Feidiou Street 18
Athens, **Greece**
Phone: 30-1/362 9717

Diabetes Division, Society for the Study
of Endocrinology, Metabolism and
Reproduction
Department of Medicine
University of Hong Kong
Pokfulam Road, **Hong Kong**
Phone 1: 852-3/855 1143

Hungarian Diabetes Association
Korányi S. u. 2a
Budapest 1083, **Hungary**
Phone: 36-1/330-360
Telex: 226161 VESEO-H

Diabetic Association of India
Maneckji Wadia Building
1st Floor, 127 M.G. Road
Bombay 400001, **India**
Phone 1: 91-22/27 38 13
Phone 2: 91-22/46 75 69(70)

Iranian Diabetes Society
1-37 Varshow St.
Behjatabad, Tehran, 15987, **Iran**
Phone 1: 98-21/89 99 21
Phone 2: 98-21/65 05 06

Irish Diabetic Association
82/83 Lr. Gardiner Street
Dublin 1, **Ireland**
Phone: 363022

Israel Diabetes Association
17 Ranak Street
Tel Aviv 63464, **Israel**
Phone 1: 972-3/5440129
Phone 2; 972-3/232274

Associazione Italiana per
la Difesa Degli Interesi di Diabetici
Via del Scrofa 14
Roma, Italy
Phone: 39-2/654 3784

National Federation of Diabetes
Associations
Via Rucellai, 46/8
20126 Milano, **Italy**
Phone 1: 39-2/5458405
Phone 2: 39-2/2578883

Italian Diabetology Society
Istituto di Patologia Speciale Med.
Universita di Perugia
Via E. Dal Pozza
06100 Perugia, **Italy**
Phone: 39-75/21.366, 23.623

Japan Diabetes Society
Hongo Sky Building 403
3-38-11 Hongo
Bunkyo-ku, Tokyo 113, **Japan**
Phone: 81-3/815 4364
Telefax: 81-3/815 7985

Kenya Diabetic Association
P.O. Box 55098
Nairobi, **Kenya**
254-5/336-725
254-5/340-740

Korean Diabetes Association
Room 603
The Korean Medical Association Building
302-75, Ichon Dong, Yongsan Ku
Séoul, 140-030, **Republic of Korea**

Association Luxembourgeoise du Diabète
P.O. Box 1316
Luxembourg
Grand-Duché de Luxembourg
Phone: 352/474545, 4411-1

L'Association Malgache contre le Diabète
P.O. Box 3097
Antananarivo 101, **Madagascar**
Phone 1: 261-2/293 63
Phone 2: 261-2/223 84

Malaysian Diabetes Association
Room 2, 5th Floor
Bangunan MMA
124 Jalan Pahang
53000 Kuala Lumpur, **Malaysia**
Phone: 60-3/44 16498
Telex: UKM 31496

Diabetes Association (Malta)
P.O. Box 413
Valletta, **Malta**
Phone 1: 356/674879
Phone 2: 356/443340

Mauritius Diabetic Association
c/o P.O. Box 17
Rose Hill, **Mauritius**
Phone 1: 230/2-4155
Phone 2: 230/2-4053
Telex: 4325 KAILASH IW

Mexican Diabetes Association
Calz. del Valle 400 local 17
Apartado Postal 52
Garza García, N.L. 66200, **Mexico**
Phone 1: 52-83/358 708
Phone 2: 52-83/564 987
Telefax: 52-83/358 708

Mexican Society of Nutrition and
Endocrinology
Vasco de Quiroga No. 15, Tlalpan
Mexico, D.F. 1400, **Mexico**
Phone: 52-5/73 12 00 ext. 2303

Dutch Diabetes Association
Puntenburgerlaan 91
3812 CC, Amersfoort
Postbus 933, 3800 AX Amersfoort,
The Netherlands
Phone: 31-33/63 05 66
Telefax: 31-33/63 09 30

Diabetic Association of Curacao
Alexanderlaan 10
Willemstad
Curacao, **Netherlands Antilles**

Dutch Association for Diabetes Research
De Boelelaan 1117
1081 HV Amsterdam, **The Netherlands**

Diabetes New Zealand Inc.
4 Coquet Street
P.O. Box 54
Oamaru, South Island, **New Zealand**
Phone: 64-3/434 8100
Telefax: 64-3/434 5281

Diabetic Association of Nigeria
39, Ogunlana Drive
Surulere, Lagos, **Nigeria**
Phone: 234-1/830 762

Norwegian Diabetes Association
Østensjøvn. 29
0661 Oslo 6, **Norway**
Phone: 47-2/65 45 50
Telefax: 47-2/63 06 88

Diabetic Association of Pakistan
5-E/3, Nazimabad, Paposhnagar
Karachi, 74600, **Pakistan**
Phone: 92-21/616890
Telex: 23507 TAZAM PK

Panamanian Diabetes Association
Apartado 957
Calle 34 y 36, Ave. Mexico
Panamá 1, **Panama**
Phone 1: 507/27-4122
Phone 2: 507/25-6372
Telex: HOSPITOMAS

Paraguayian Society of Diabetology
Coronel Moreno 1030
Asuncion, **Paraguay**
Phone 1: 595-21/604-499
Phone 2: 595-21/98-032
Telefax: 595-21/44 8036

Peruvian Society of Endocrinology
Casilla 435
Lima, **Peru**

Peruvian Diabetes Association
Apartado 106
Lima 1, **Peru**
Phone: 51/31-1333, 72-1095

Philippine Diabetes Association
Room 304, Polymedic General Hospital
163 E. de los Santos Avenue
Mandaluyong
Metro Manilla, **Philippines**
Phone: 63-2/70.75.21, 79.91.56

Polish Diabetological Association
Kopernika 17
31-501 Kraków
Kraków, **Poland**
Phone 1: 48-12/21 01 44
Phone 2: 48-12/21-40-54

Portuguese Diabetic Association
Rua do Salitre, 118
1200 Lisbon, **Portugal**
Phone 1: 351-1/680041(42)
Phone 2: 351-2/682729

Puerto Rican Society of Endocrinology
and Diabetology
P.O. Box 41174 Estación Minillas
San Juan, **Puerto Rico** 00940

Unión des Societés des Sciences
Medicales
de la République Socialiste de Roumanie
8 Rue Progresulul B.P. 190
70754 Bucharest, **Romania**
Phone: 40-0/14 10 71

Saudi Diabetes and
Endocrine Association
P.O. Box 1498
Al Khobar 31952, **Saudi Arabia**
Phone: 966-3/826-2111
Telex: 801636 AFHOSP SJ
Telefax: 966-3/827-4747

Diabetic Society of Singapore
11 Penang Lane # 03-03/04
Singapore Council of Social
Service Building
Orchard Point, P.O. Box 82
Singapore 9123, **Republic of
Singapore** 0923
Phone: 65/3373971

Society for Endocrinology,
Metabolism and Diabetes of Southern
Africa (SEMDSA)
P.O. Box 783155
Sandton 2146
Johannesburg, **South Africa**
Phone: 27-11/7837275

South African Diabetes Association
Room 51, 5th Floor, Cuthberts Building
12 Plein Street
Cape Town, 8001, **South Africa**
Phone: 27-21/461-3715
Telefax: 27-21/462-2008

Spanish Diabetes Society
Colegio Oficial de Médicos
Santa Isabel, 51
28012 Madrid, **Spain**

Diabetic Association of Sri Lanka
102 Barnes Place
Colombo 7, **Sri Lanka**
Phone: 94-1/93 375

Sudan Diabetic Association
P.O. Box 102
c/o Faculty of Medicine
University of Khartoum
Khartoum, **Sudan**
Phone: 249-11/722 24

Stichting Diabetes Suriname
Gravenstraat 7 bo
Paramaribo, **Suriname**
Phone: 597/743-47

Swedish Society of Endocrinology
Department of Internal Medicine
University Hospital
S-751 85 Uppsala, **Sweden**
Phone: 46-18/663000

Swedish Diabetes Association
P.O. Box 1545
179 29 Solna, **Sweden**
Phone 1: 46-8/29 60 00
Telefax: 46-8/98 25 25

Swiss Diabetes Association
Hegarstrasse 18
CH-8032 Zurich, **Switzerland**
Phone: 41-1/383 13 15
Telefax: 41-1/55 89 12

Chinese Taipei Diabetes Association
No. 1, Chang-Te Street
Taipei, Taiwan 10016, **Taiwan**
Phone 1: 886-2/312-3456 ext. 2212
Phone 2: 886-2/396-0283

Diabetic Association for Thailand
Mongkutkao Hospital, Payatai
Bangkok, **Thailand**
Phone: 66-2464061

Tunisian Diabetic Association
3, Rue El Moaskar
Tunis 1000, **Tunisia**
Phone: 216-1/254-399

Turkish Diabetes Association
Osmanbey, Safak Sokak No. 44
Daire 2
Istanbul, **Turkey**
Phone: 91-1/148 55 23, 148 60 86

Uganda Diabetic Association
Department of Medicine
Makerere University
P.O. Box 7072 Mulago Hospital
Kampala, **Uganda**
Phone: 256-41/54001

British Diabetic Association
10 Queen Anne Street
London W1M 0BD, **United Kingdom**
Phone: 44-1/323-1531
Telefax: 44-1/637-3644

American Diabetes Association
1660 Duke Street
Alexandria, VA 22314,
United States of America
Phone 1: 1-703/549-1500
Phone 2: 1-800/232-3472 (USA Only)
Telex: 901132 ADA ALE
Telefax: 1-703/836-7439

Uruguayan Diabetes Association
Paraguay 1273
Montevideo, **Uruguay**

Phone 1: 598-2/91-62-14
Phone 2: 598-2/98-39-79

Venezuelan Endocrinology and
Metabolism Society
Edificio Fundavac
Av. Neveri, Colinas de Bello Monte
P.O. Box 61843
Caracas 1041-A, **Venezuela**
Phone 1: 58-2/751 37 68
Phone 2: 58-2/62 11 33

Venezuelan Diabetes Association
Av. Caracas 464
Barquisimeto, **Venezuela**
Phone: 58/525373

The Association of Diabetic Societies
of Yugoslavia
4a Dugi Dol, P.O. Box 958
41000 Zagreb, **Yugoslavia**
Phone 1: 38-41/232 222
Phone 2: 38-41/231-480
Telex: INDIAB 22353

Provisional Members

Bahrain Diabetes Association
P.O. Box 12
Salmaniya Medical Centre, **Bahrain**
Telex: 8881
Telefax: 669166

Iraqi Diabetes Association
Head of Department of Medicine
Faculty of Medicine
Al-Mostansereya University
P.O. Box 14132
Baghdad, **Iraq**

Mozambican Diabetes Association
C.P. 2167
Maputo, **Mozambique**

Swedish Society for Diabetology
Akademiska Sjukhuset
751 85 Uppsala, **Sweden**
Phone: 46-18/66 30 00
Telefax: 46-18/55 31 04

Diabetes Association of
Trinidad and Tobago
P.O. Box 1095
Port-of-Spain, **Trinidad**, W.I.
Phone: 1-809/662-8161, 662-4843
Telefax: 1-809/642-2584

Zambia Diabetic Association
P.O. Box 35365
Lusaka, **Zambia**
Phone: (01) 250 110
